Foreword

Because I'm far from being a "traditional" individual, this

book comes in 3 parts; the 1st part being a focus on

achieving your maximum health potential with focuses on

the mental, physical, and emotional aspects of said health.

The 2nd part is focused on helping you become your own

fitness snob and attain your perfect health through proper

thinking and fitness programming.

The 3rd part is focused on eating to achieve your optimal

health and vitality levels. This focuses on the energetic

aspects of the food you eat to help you make informed

choices.

Enjoy, and read OFTEN!!

Dedication

I dedicate this book to my wife, who put up with my nagging and 2am creativity sessions, my son Blake, who taught me that it IS possible to bond with your baby and type legible words with your left hand, friends, family, and everyone in the world, in hopes that they will feel a powerful hunger inside every time they pick up this tome, to grow healthier and more vital and help the entire planet in so doing.

God Bless!

PART 1

Master Keys to Health and Vitality!!

The techniques in this manual are not intended to treat or cure anything. If you have a health issue, then please consult with the proper individuals. When practicing the breathing meditation exercises, please do NOT perform while driving or operating heavy machinery.

Before you jump right in and start using these techniques, I want you to realize something very important: the more you practice (read: use) these techniques, the easier it becomes for your body to relax in ANY situation to the point where you feel as though you can fall asleep ANYWHERE.

If you're reading this now, then chances are you want to find ways to deal with the stresses that occur in your everyday life. That's natural. It's natural for us to want to find ways to deal with the challenges in our life.

Stress is one of those challenges or more specifically, learning to deal with stress. We all deal with it in our own unique way. When some people get stressed out, they get angry. When some people get stressed out, they get scared. Some people eat. Some people don't eat. The reactions to stress are as varied as the types of people there are in the world today, but one thing is certain: That's a hell of a lot of reactions!!!

Do you realize that almost every illness is STRESS RELATED?? Are you starting to see how when you learn to how relax you can help yourself avoid all those nasty stress related illnesses?

One thing that you need to realize is this: Stress is a part of life. Stress is universal. Stress is timeless. Alexander The great was stressed out. At the time of this writing, President Obama gets stressed out. You get stressed out. Your friends and family get stressed out. There's not a living being on this great big blue earth that doesn't get stressed out.

Hanz Seyle, A Vienna born Hungarian scientist, spent his life studying stress – specifically what it is and its effect upon living beings ("people" for the lay person…)☺. He coined the terms "Stress" and "Fight or Flight Response". Seyle defined stress as "the nonspecific response of the body to any demand". It encompasses all physical and psychological reactions to the demands placed upon the individual by his internal and his external environments. Without stress, progress in life is not possible. Stress is completely normal and cannot be avoided. Seyle makes the distinction between EUSTRESS and DISTRESS. According to Seyle, Eustress is produced by doing what we LIKE TO DO and what is good for us. Distress is elicited by those activities and situations that we DON'T LIKE TO DO, but we must. Can you think of any activities that you don't like to do? Can you think of all the activities that you like to do? Can you sense the reactions you have to both types of activities and situations? Can you see how simply thinking about the things you like to do, and don't like to, can cause you to feel a certain way?

Did you know that weight lifting can elicit the stress response in people? When a person first begins a weight training program, their body usually isn't used to the strain place upon the muscles by the external force, in this case, the weight. However, within a few weeks, the body has adapted and repaired itself and is able to handle the stressor (the weight) without adverse side effects, i.e. muscle soreness. So now, A 20 pound weight that a person could only curl 8 times becomes child's play and now the person can lift that weight 20 times easily!!! Now, what do you think is going to happen to that person's muscles when they attempt to lift a 25 pound weight for the 1st time? The stress response, of course!!! It's a new stressor or to put it more productively, it's a new stimulus. So the entire body will need to adapt to the extra weight. The skeletal system, the circulatory system, the cardiovascular system, all of them.

When you understand that the body is in a constant state of change and that many forces, both internal and external, are constantly influencing our physical and emotional states of being, then you'll find it easier to understand the stress response and how important it is to daily life.

Yes, I said important. If you don't have the capacity to adapt, then you would never adapt to the challenges in your life and therefore, you would never grow. In fact, in all likelihood, you would back slide. Remember, life is in constant motion and if you're not advancing, then you'll stay the same, if you're lucky...

The cool thing about stress that Seyle discovered was that every living being has a three phase reaction to stress, which he called the Generalized Adaptation Syndrome:

1)   Alarm Reaction: In this first phase, the reaction of the body to stress is an "alarm reaction" in which the ability to respond temporarily decreases. This is a kind of shock reaction that is usually of short duration.

2)   State of Resistance: If stress continues, extra cortisone and adrenaline are produced and released, increasing the body's ability to adapt to the stress and improve performance of the activities required by the stressor. This adaptation to the stressor results in a sharpening of the senses, an increase in the precision of motor control of the body, increased wakefulness and alertness, and a high metabolic rate. This results in increased performance of the activities carried

out at this time. If the stress still does not stop, the quantity of these chemicals in the bloodstream increases until the body reaches its peak of ability to react to the stress. Seyle calls this the "state of resistance". This keeps the organism able to react swiftly and powerfully. This is a wise reaction of the body that promotes survival in conditions of extended stress. How long the body can support this process is individual.

3)   State Of Exhaustion – When this state of resistance continues too long, there comes what Seyle calls the "state of exhaustion". When more or less completely exhausted, the body cannot produce the extra chemicals and energy for further resistance. The reserves are used up. In common phraseology, this is referred to "burn out". In this state, rest, therapy, good nutrition and a change of lifestyle are desperately needed for the body (and mind) to be relieved from stress and to recover from the exhausted state.

Seyle found the following symptoms to be typically associated with stress:

- Recurring infections

- Allergies and hay fever

- Stomach and other digestive symptoms

- Insomnia, irritability, lack of energy, unusual mental symptoms

- Lack of concentration, confusion of thought

- Chronic fatigue, depressive tendencies

- Trembling, Nervous tics, stuttering

- Teeth grinding at night, leading to a greater sensitivity to sweet/sour, hot/cold

- Diarrhea

- Migraine, premenstrual syndrome

- Neck and Back Pain

- Too great or too small an appetite

- A strong or even addictive desire for nicotine, alcohol, coffee, or other stimulants/drugs

Do you have any of the symptoms of stress that Seyle observed? Can you think of any of your friends and family that are constantly stating that they have these symptoms?

Seyle's research led him to develop a guideline for health through the reduction of Distress and finding more activities that provide a source of Eustress. He also came to the conclusion that to promote health, the best attitude and lifestyle for all living beings is "altruistic egotism". He coined the phrase as an alternative to the nearly impossible recommendation of Jesus Christ to "love thy neighbor as thyself". I'm pretty sure it is possible for some people, but not for me, not right now…

For Selye, altruistic egotism implies that being benevolent to others promotes self preservation. Interpret that however you like. This means that the best way to be assured that others will help you when you need them is to help them when they need you.

Here are a few of Seyle's recommendations:

- Find your own natural stress level. In other words, determine how much stress you can put with before you just stand up, throw off all your clothes, and run down the street butt naked screaming "enough is enough!!"
- Learn the difference between eustress and distress

- Precisely analyze your problems. Look at the situation as it is.

- Don't force and overexert yourself. Rather, learn to know and follow your own need for rest and relaxation. Pay attention to your body and listen to the messages it's sending you.

- Avoid one side stresses. The body wants to balance one kind of stress like hard physical work with another kind of stress like reading or making music.

- Observe your "stress quotient" with relation to your specific stress and general stress. When there is too much specific stress, one needs to get involved in other kinds of activities. Specific stress is what it's called when the stress response is elicited in a specific context or certain situation i.e. in the workplace. When there is too much general stress, one needs rest and relaxation in a quiet non-stressing environment. General stress is just what it sounds like - when you get stressed out by seemingly simple occurrences.

As if this wasn't enough, Seyle's research indicates that stress weakens the immune system, whose job it is to recognize and fight against undesirable substances in the body, like viruses and such. Since immune system weakness is the root of many of todays most prevalent and difficult medical problems, a deeper consideration of seyle's concepts by medical doctors and other health professionals is worth noting. The relationship between stress and disease is very powerful and we need to take stress into consideration when we talk about illness.

I love Seyle's idea of a "Stress Quotient". Essentially, a stress quotient is a subjective of your stress levels. How stressed out do you feel, on a scale of 1 – 10 (or any other numbers that you feel comfortable using)? Is there a certain level of stress that you can reach before your performance starts to suffer for it? Is it a 5? Is it a 9? What's your stress quotient? This is very important to become aware of.

A simple way to get an idea of your Individual Stress Quotient is to notice how good you feel when you first wake up in the morning, after a night of relaxing, refreshing sleep. This feeling that you feel is going to be your "baseline" mood. We can't compare things unless we have something to measure against, right?

We need a CONTROL, which is going to be your feeling of wellbeing first thing in the morning. Depending on the night before however, this can be relative… to make things a little easier, after you read the following instructions, you're going to put this book down, do the drills, and then you going to pick up this book and keep reading. Sounds like a plan, right? Here goes:

1) Remember a time when you felt really relaxed. Remember a time when you felt like you had all the time in the world and you felt really good. Remember what you saw; remember what you heard, remember how you felt. Really relive that moment. As you remember that now, really allow those feelings to grow and expand and fill your mind and body.

2) Now… Remember a time when you felt really stressed out. Remember what you heard, remember what you saw, and remember what you felt. Really relive that moment. Really allow those feelings to be as strong as they were when you first felt them.

Now, you may be wondering "what the hell was the purpose of that?!?!??" Well, the little exercise above serves two purposes: The first exercise is designed to help you change your state of being to a more relaxed state. The second exercise is designed to help you remember what it's like to be stressed out. Now, why would anyone want to remember what it's like to be stressed out? Well…

You have to know how you're feeling before you change the way you feel.

Doesn't that make sense? You have to be aware that there is something to change before you can change it. Think of it as having radar: if a certain object isn't on your radar, then how can you notice it? Do you get the picture now?

Stress can be a good thing, when you stop and think about it. The frustration and anger you feel can be directed towards the accomplishment of your goals. Those stressful emotions are the things that you no longer want to feel. Think of your goals as the destination. Now, think of your body as the vehicle. Now, think of your emotions as the fuel for the vehicle. Use your emotions as

16

fuel to push you toward your goals and desires. Use your dreams and desires to pull you towards what it is you do want to have and experience. That's part of the function of emotions. Our emotions are much like signals. Good feelings let us know that we're doing something right. Bad feelings like boredom or fear let us know that something is wrong and something needs to be changed. If you're stressed out about a situation, it's obvious that you need to do something to change the situation in your favor, isn't it? If you can change your situation so that it's much better, then doesn't it make perfect sense that you want to do that, not only for your financial situation, but for your health as well?

When you take the time to figure out what it is that you DO WANT, then you can blast toward it at the speed of life.

Now...

According to Donna Eden, author of "Energy Medicine for Women", there's something very interesting about the way men and women respond to stress:

"...When a woman faces stress, her body produces oxytocin, which buffers the fight or flight response and causes her to seek ways of connecting with others. Whatever way she decides on, is totally up to her. After any immediate threat, her focus goes to conferring with other women and tending to the welfare of the children. The more she does this, the more oxytocin she produces..."

Men, on the other hand:

"... Testosterone, on the other hand, which men produce in high levels when stressed, tends to inhibit the bonding effects of oxytocin. When relationships become strained, most women want to talk; most men turn inward and seek solutions in isolation..."

If you look back at your experiences, I think you'll find examples in which the above is accurate.

Another reason you want to learn ways to neutralize the stress response is because stress causes your body to release small amounts of a chemical called Cortisol. You may have seen infomercials offering supplements which are designed to block the release of that chemical. While I don't necessarily agree with them if cortisol is so bad, then why does your body produce it? Does it make sense that nature would give us the ability to produce cortisol if it didn't offer us some benefit?), the main point is that cortisol can contribute to excess weight gain. My main issue with cortisol blockers is that they are focused on the SYMPTOMS and not the CAUSE. There's a cause to your stress, and when you address the cause, you address the effect, understand? Do you think it's easier to put out a fire by dowsing water on top of it, or do you think it's easier to put out a fire by aiming at the base?

So, when dealing with stress, you want to start at the CAUSE. Really ask yourself:

"What is causing me to be/feel stressed out?"

And most importantly:

"What about this situation is causing me to be stressed out?"

One simple way to neutralize or at least reduce the intensity of the stress your feeling in relation to a specific context/situation is to change the way you view the situation. When you change the way you look at the situation, you change the way you react to it. You can change the way you view a situation by putting it into its proper context: Realize that the situation will only change when YOU change it and when you get through this thing you're dealing with to the other side, life will be better and you will be better for having experienced this. Stop and ask yourself: Is this a situation that I change? If so, how can I change this situation so that I actually enjoy it?

How can you change your own beliefs and attitudes so that the environment which sucked now provides you a challenge which you can use to build your spiritual muscles up until you find/create an environment that's perfect for you?

If you could create the perfect environment for you, what would you create?

I like to look at life as a sort of road trip. The final destination being the purpose that we were born to fulfill. The problems that we experience being little stumbling blocks or detours that can make us lose sight of the final destination. In the story of your life, is this challenge you're dealing with going to earn a footnote? I feel like we all have a purpose to fulfill in life. Finding it is not so much the challenge; it's allowing yourself to actually let go and live your purpose that seems to be this major issue with some people. How do you look at life?

Really ask yourself this question: "Am I perceiving this situation to be bigger than it actually is?

Keep in mind that this little process will help eliminate the stress around the problem. However, it won't eliminate the problem itself. That's where you come in. You have to think of all the ways you can handle this challenge. When you come up with some ideas that you can work with, take action on them. They're only ideas until you start to see if they work or not; when you start to take action on them, then you get feedback as to what works and what doesn't.

Speaking of changing your perspective…. Did you know that your eyes hold a really amazing relaxation secret? Well, I'll tell you: There are two types of vision that people normally use, however we seem to use one more than the other. Foveal vision, or narrow focus vision is what we normally use when we're reading, or writing, of focusing on something very interesting to us. Peripheral vision is basically seeing from the left or right of your visual field without moving your eyes. Peripheral vision is mainly used for detecting movement. This form of vision is highly developed in animals for the simple fact that their survival depends upon it. If a deer doesn't see me sneaking up on it, then it's veal. See my point? Here's the really interesting thing about these two modes of seeing:

When you start to focus on your peripheral vision, you automatically turn on your parasympathetic nervous system, which is associated with relaxation and calmness. In other words, you automatically begin to **RELAX** !!!!!

In the Hawaiian spiritual practice of Huna, this form of seeing is called Hakalau. In Neuro Linguistic Programming, this state of relaxed awareness is called The Learning State. You can easily start to use your peripheral vision and relax INSTANTLY and Expand Your Awareness wherever you are:

1) Find a spot in front of you a few inches above eye level. A few inches are fine, because you don't want to strain your

eyes trying to look up at the ceiling when you only need to look at the wall ahead of you.

2) Once you're gently focused on that spot, start to allow your awareness to spread out and notice what's going on to the left and right of you. If it's too difficult for you to notice both side simultaneously, then pick one side for now and focus on that. Once you're awareness starts to become more "flexible, you'll notice that you'll start to pick up all the movements going on around you.

3) Stay there and notice what's going on in your peripheral vision for as long as it feels good. You'll notice that you start to breathe deeper and feel calmer.

4) As you in this relaxed state of being, start to notice the sounds around you. Just relax and allow your visual awareness to notice what's going on around you.

You'll want to play around with this process so that you can get the hang of it. Before you know it, you'll be automatically entering the relaxed learning state, disengage your stress response and start to think more clearly.

Now...

I'm a firm believer in the saying:

"Before you can control a thing, You Must Understand it..."

That makes perfect sense, don't you think?

Before you could EASILY drive your car down the street (for the most part), you had become familiar with all of it functions and its capabilities, which requires practice, doesn't it? You had to get used to the speed at which the car was capable of moving. You had to learn when and how to press on the brakes.

Well, learning how to handle stress is the same way: You have to understand and become aware of what happens to YOU when you get stressed out so you can take the appropriate actions to handle, so that now you...

Move from Stress to Bliss.

The techniques presented here will allow you to move from feeling stressed out and trigger happy to feeling calm and centered. The idea here is to help you develop a calm emotional state from which you can move in your daily life... so now when people see you coming around the corner, they don't run anymore. They actually want to be around you. The funny thing about emotional states is that....

They Are Contagious.

Have you ever been excited just talking with someone else who was excited? What was that like?

Have you ever been in a room full of people laughing and joking, and even though you were in a not so productive mood, you started to cheer up as you could hear the people around you laughing manically?

Hows about this then....

Have you ever been to a funeral? Have you noticed what it's like in a room full of grieving people? If you've ever been to a festive funeral, then please forgive the above example.

What's the difference between being at a funeral and being in a room full of happy people?

Using the techniques here will help you to develop your own Emotional Background Noise (tm). Think of the EBN as the song that quietly playing the background. What kind of music do YOU want playing in the background of YOUR life? It's your choice….

Do you want Death Metal Constantly Pumping?

Or do you want Mozart and Beethoven quietly rocking you in blissful awareness as you deal with the things in your life?

Once you master the principles here, you'll be able to CHOOSE which Emotional Background Noise you want to carry with you. Isn't that awesome? One simple way you can energize yourself and consequently have a positive impact on the people you interact with is to do THE THYMUS THUMP.

For those of you who don't already know, the thymus is a small gland located in the center of your chest in between your pectoral muscles. It's located right behind the sternum.

The thymus gland is one of the "arms" of your immune system, and is responsible in part for producing various antibodies like t cells, and other antibodies responsible for defending us from foreign invaders. In some respects, our immune system is like the military, and its duty is to protect its country (your body) from foreign invaders (germs and other not so nice organisms).

The thing about the thymus gland is that it tends to shrink with age. That shrinkage is associated with a decrease in your bodies' ability to ward off outside invaders.

You can easily activate your thymus gland and balance your immune system by tapping that spot right over your thymus gland about 20-30 times as your breath deeply in through the nose and out through the mouth. This is a good way to recharge yourself and start the day on a good note.

Just a word of caution: when first start to thump your thymus, you may feel some soreness in that area. Please be aware that it is not from the thumping. If you really need it, the soreness will be present, but in a few days, it'll go away never to return. I've seen people who gently slap that area have soreness the next day. The general rule of thumb with any type of self massage is:

If it hurts, then your body needs it!!!

The good thing about this little process is that you can do it anytime you want, anywhere you want. Just don't do it in front of your boss. Or in front of your loved ones. Don't do it in front of people period. Unless you want to explain to them what you're doing and why you're doing it. Of course, if you want to do it in front of people, and they ask you where you learned it, then you can go ahead and tell them☺

Now...

Another technique that I like to use is called the EAR TUG. It's a technique used in acupressure to help relax the body and release stress. The ears have many acupressure points on them and when you stimulate your ears, you can stimulate and relax your body. To perform this technique, all you have to do is – surprise, surprise – pull and tug on your ears. GENTLY tug and pull on your ears, because they are sensitive. If you rip your ears off, then you're probably doing it too rough… and I'm not responsible for that. For those of you not familiar with meridians and how they work, and for the sake of time and understanding, there's a major meridian that flows along the ears, and when you tug and pull on your ears GENTLY, you release any energy that has become congested along that meridian, and at the same time, you release stress.
Now…

What if I told you that stress can be a good thing? You may be thinking "Amir, those two words don't even look like they belong together in the same sentence, sort of like some people in thongs..."

Let's talk about what happens in the body when we undergo the stress response. Whenever we get stressed out, we undergo something called "The fight or Flight response". It is a profound set of changes that occur whenever we are faced with a stressful or threatening situation. This response prepares the body for a PHYSICAL REACTION to a real or perceived threat - to fight or to run away.

Here are some of the physiological changes associated with it:

- Metabolism Increases

- Heart rate increases

- Blood pressure Increases

- Breathing Rate Increases

- Muscle Tension Increases

All of these changes are the result of adrenaline and noradrenalin being released into your bloodstream. Your vision might narrow a bit so that you go from using peripheral vision to tunnel vision, which can further enhance the fight or flight response. If you see can't anything around you and you're extremely terrified, what do think will happen?

With the fight or Flight Response, the name of the game is AROUSAL. It's designed to make you alert so you can handle the perceived threat. I would think it's very hard to run from a grizzly bear if you're completely relaxed, don't you?

Notice that I said the word "Perceived".

Well, what's that mean? It means that even if the stress or situation is IMAGINED, the body still reacts by undergoing the Fight Or flight response. This demonstrates the connection between the Mind and the Body. What you think about or imagine vividly and repeatedly is reflected in your body. If you're a guy or a gal and you're a human being, then I don't have to tell you what it's like when you think about your dream guy or gal in that… special way, do I?

It means that just sitting there and thinking about that upcoming interview is enough to activate the response. Just sitting there and thinking about dealing with "person A" or "person B" is enough to have you grinding your teeth and reaching for your baseball bat.

30

It means that just sitting there and thinking about that date with the chick from accounting is enough to activate the response.

It means just thinking about what happened last week is enough to trigger the response.

Now....

This response is perfect when you're camping in the woods and a Giant-normous (my very own word) Black Bear Jumps out of a tree and wants your honey... In that case, you want to be as fast as possible (actually, in that case, they say that you shouldn't run because then the bear will chase you down like a member of the Buffalo Bills Defense...). You want that response when you're walking down the street at night and there's someone that's been walking too close to you for too long...

However....

Do you think it's a good thing to undergo that response for something like driving in Rush Hour traffic, an everyday occurrence? Probably not.

So, right about now, you're probably saying to yourself,"

What can I do to stop the response from happening?" The bad news is that you can't. The good news is that there is another response that we undergo, called The Relaxation Response.

The Relaxation Response was discovered By Dr. Herbert Benson, who found it while doing research with practitioners of Transcendental Meditation. He discovered a set of physiological responses that accompanied relaxation:

"... We all found that several major physiological systems responded to the simple act of sitting quietly and giving the mind a focus; the metabolism decreased; the heart rate slowed; respiratory rate decreased, and there were distinctive brain waves(alpha brainwaves)..."

We all undergo the Relaxation Response, whether we realize it or not. When you're sitting at home or in your favorite place with your favorite book and favorite drink in each hand, and you sigh deeply... You're undergoing the Relaxation Response.

When you're standing in your favorite spot and you looking at an amazing view, you're body is beginning to relax deeply...

When you have your arms wrapped around someone that

you care about and you know that this person really cares about you, you relax completely. In fact, scientific studies have demonstrated that physical contact has the ability to speed up the rate at which a person heals from injuries. There's a complete practice utilizing touch and intention could "Therapeutic Touch". There's some very fascinating stuff there and it's worth a closer look by the medical community. If it works, when are YOU going to start using it?

Another thing that I noticed and really like about therapeutic touch is the use of centering techniques before they apply their skills in healing another. The technique they use is to relax… and visualize an object, preferably something natural that causes you to relax when you think about it. What natural places do you enjoy being in? Whatever it is, bring it to mind and focus on that for awhile. When you focus on something that relaxes or makes you feel good, you mind sort resonates to that image and surprise, surprise…. You automatically induce the relaxation response!!!
Now...

You know About the Various responses that the body undergoes in response to Stress and Relaxation. You may be wondering: "How can I induce the Relaxation Response anytime I please?"

That's a very good question, the answer to which will change your life - And the life of those you hangs out with everyday - for the better. Remember earlier how I mentioned that emotional States are contagious? Well...

Which do you prefer: A sunny, vibrant day filled with excitement or a cloudy, somber day, which is damp and cold?

Anyway…

Another very simple way to relax and trigger your relaxation response is to laugh your ass off. Surprise, surprise, right? We all know that laughter is good for us, but how many of us actually use that knowledge and force ourselves to piss our pants laughing? Not too many people, I have to say. Can you remember a time when you laughed so hard that every muscle in your face ached and your stomach felt like Arnold Schwarzenegger just gave you a massage? Can you remember what you saw? Can you remember what you heard? As you remember that incident. Now, allow yourself to fully relive that experience. Automatically, you'll start to smile to yourself as you think about that time.

Now...

Imagine what it will be like when you're completely at ease and you're interacting with the people you deal with everyday. Imagine how they'll respond to you when you're in that relaxed state. Do you think they'll want to be around you more?

I think so. In fact...

I know so!!!

When I'm pissed off, I'm not good to be around. However, when I realize that I'm pissed off and I use the principles here to change that so that now I'm relaxed, everybody wants to be around me. I'm sure it's the same thing with you.

Now....

The most important thing to realize here is that in order for you to relax completely, you have to make the DECISION that you are going to relax. It's okay to WANT to relax, and it's even better to RELAX. The intention to RELAX is the most important thing. We all have our own little relaxation rituals:

Some people Smoke

Some people have a drink or two.

Some People make love. Good lovemaking will melt the tensest

persons'...um, tension. You know the feeling you get after having

really athletic sex?

Some people take a warm bath.

These little rituals work because of the INTENTION to relax.

Intention is very powerful and scientific research has PROVEN that

intention can influence the mind and body.

One of the most important things about a ritual is that you

need to find a sacred space. You need to dedicate a place to

relaxation and letting loose. Where ever that place may be, make

sure the only thing that goes on there is total relaxation and

vegetation.

When you're in your sacred space, cell phones and memos

mean absolutely nothing. You can forget all about them and focus your attention on yourself and the relaxation of your body.

Your sacred space of relaxation can be ANYWHERE you feel relaxed. ANYWHERE.

In a nutshell, you sacred space is a physical location in that you associate with relaxation. This can be ANYWHERE, even a certain spot on the ground that you stand and suddenly, your body is completely relaxed. In neuron linguistic programming, the process of associating desired states with physical locations around you is called Spatial Anchoring. Incredibly effective speakers and effective politicians make use of Spatial Anchoring strategically. In a nutshell, they talk about good, positive, uplifting topics in one spot, and they talk about, rotten, nasty, disgusting things while they are standing in another location. When they want their audience to associate someone or something with general dirtbagged-ness (my own word, just created), they will go back to that location where they discussed and elicited negative reactions and talk about their competitors. I wonder how many politicians have done that..... Naw, it is not possible... So, how can you, being the intelligent and career minded person that you are, use this little tactic to your advantage? I bet you sure didn't expect to get a little lesson in Covert influence while reading a guide on Stress reduction and Relaxation did you? There are many good sources that give complete instructions on how to use spatial anchoring.

You get the idea, don't you?

Another thing to keep in mind is that we are all different in many ways, including the ways in which we like to recharge our batteries. Some people like to go out and get wild and some people like to stay in and take a nap. No one way of recharging is better than the other, except in each person's own life. Which way do you choose to recharge your batteries:

Interaction or Introspection?

One way you can relax completely and even fix your vision a little bit is when you use a process called "Palming". It's not what you're thinking about, but that definitely helps you relax. "Palming" is a technique used by an English doctor by the name of William Bates. He discovered that eyes need complete rest in order to fix themselves. By complete rest, he means that the eyes need to take a break from any stimulus. The eyes main stimulus is light. When you rub your palms and put them over your eyes, you prevent light from hitting the eyes and thus you provide the eyes with complete rest. Think of this palming procedure like this: when you lie down in bed, and close your eyes, the next thing you know, it's the next morning or week or whatever, and you're fully refreshed and you're ready to go out into the world. When you palm, you allow your eyes to go to sleep and rest so they can wake refreshed and ready to take in all the information around you. Now, I don't know if you realize this or not, but the eyes are one of our primary ways of sensing the world around us. Doesn't it make sense that you want them to be working as perfectly as possible?

You can palm anywhere you can find time to be alone and undisturbed. As you sit there with your palms over your eyes, you can practice visualizing different things and activities. Are you planning something special for this weekend? Why don't you go ahead and mentally rehearse it as you're palming!!!
If you do prefer to sleep in and rejuvenate yourself, then...

Allow the outside world to gradually MELT AWAY for NOW. Your problems and obligations will be there when you're ready to deal with them. In your sacred place of relaxation, you're only obligation is to YOURSELF and your total relaxation. The basic formula is:

$$Relaxation = Rejuvenation$$

If you're one of those extroverted party animals that like to socialize to recharge your batteries, then do I really need to give you any advice? What I need to do is get your number so we can all party☺

When you're deeply relaxed, your muscles release unwanted tension and your allow your thoughts to roam where they will. You relinquish control for just a minute so your body can work its restorative magic. Is it any wonder why you feel good after a night of refreshing, rejuvenating sleep? When we sleep, our conscious minds seem to go somewhere, and our bodies are freed from the tensions of daily life for 6 to 8 hours. That's like a 6-8 hour relaxing massage. And on top of this, you can watch any movies you want (dreams). Doesn't sleep sound AWESOME when you think about it like that?

Now...

What do you think happens when you don't get as much sleep as your body needs? Well, being the smart person who was intelligent to get this manual, I think you can make a good guess, can't you?

Make sleep a priority in your life. Listen to your body. When you feel tired, and if it is at all possible to do so, take a nap. Scientific research has proven that when we so much as close our eyes, our brainwaves slow down from producing beta waves, which are associated with AROUSAL and they start to produce Alpha waves, which are associated with daydreaming and RELAXATION.

Another really awesome way to relax after a long hard day on your feet is to lie down in the yoga posture called "The Corpse Pose". The position sound like what it is: You lie on your back with your arms to your sides, palms up, and you allow your feet to relax completely and fall outward a bit, which they should do naturally when you're lying down like that. When you think about it, the corpse pose is a natural response to a long, hard day: you come home, you kick off your shoes, throw all your stuff in the corner, and then you plop backwards on your bed, as you allow all that tension to just…melt away.

As you lie in this posture, you can relax your body from head to toe and pay attention to any sensations that you might feel. When you notice any areas of tension, take a deep breath and release it through your mouth. When you do this, you allow that tension to just… melt away.

Another thing that I like about the corpse pose is that you can take that time to go inside and center yourself inside your body. We spend so much time with our awareness focused on the word around us, with all the stimulus from television and radio and bosses and coworkers, and so on… and isn't it nice to just focus on yourself for awhile and forget all about the outside world for a moment?

It's okay if you want to fall asleep as you lay there. The purpose of lying in this pose is COMPLETE RELAXATION. If you fall asleep, then it means that your body needs it. Don't you want to give your body what it needs?

Speaking of tension...

Many of us carry around unwanted tension in our bodies daily. We may be tense on the drive to work and not even be aware of it. We may be tense at a seemingly relaxing event or location. In other words, you may think your relaxed, when in fact, you're as tense as a wound up spring. Unnecessary tension is a waste of energy. It takes effort to tense a muscle. Now, imagine how much energy you're wasting when you are walking around tensed up without reason.

I believe that constant tension is a side effect of some fear or anxiety a person may be feeling. You ever notice the difference between the way you feel when you're walking along the country side and the way you feel when you're walking down a city street? There's a big difference there, if you take the time to notice that. Whatever the case may be, chronic unnecessary tension is a waste of energy and we need to learn relaxation techniques to counter this phenomenon, don't you agree?

Now...

People are different in where they carry chronic tension. Some people constantly carry tension in the shoulders. Some people walk around with extremely tight asses. Some people walk with clenched fists. Where do you constantly carry unnecessary tension?

A good way to dissolve any tension you may be carrying is to start to become aware of your body and how it feels from time to time. Your body can be very "loud" when it wants to get a message across. When you're sitting in a certain way for a certain length of time, and your body starts to feel a certain way, don't you feel compelled to move to a different position?

Well, what happened was your body was delivering a message, and you received it, resulting in a change in posture. This is basis of biofeedback: you hear the message, and you send your body another message. From now on, start to pay attention to the way your body feels as you are walking, exercising, or sitting. Make changes based on the way you feel. Adjust yourself until you find a position that feels good. That's the key. If it feels good, then it's good.

Another time our bodies "scream" at us is when it's in pain. It's screaming because it needs our attention to take care of the problem. Things like drugs and painkillers only mask the Effect of the cause. Take care of the problem and the pain goes away. Remember what I said earlier about taking care of the cause to eliminate the effects? Think about it, and I think you'll find that it makes perfect sense.

Have you ever heard the saying "Your body is your temple"? Well, that's true in a sense and I like to think of your body as your personal vehicle through life. Sure, you may have break downs and may hit a few bumps along the road, and when you take care of it and change the oil frequently (colon cleansing) and make sure it gets that proper fuel and usage (food and exercise), then you can keep your car (body) for a long time. Or at least until they make the first cybernetic body so we can transplant our brains into them.... anyway, you get the point, don't you?

Another good thing that will allow you to release unwanted tension is to stretch throughout the day. I don't mean a complete stretching session like the ones that I might offer to clients. I mean just standing up wherever you might be and moving your body in ways that feel good to you. Stretch your arms up to the sky as high you can. You might be surprised how your body reacts.

Stretching a muscle is sort of like wringing out a wash rag. You know how the rag gets filled with water as you take a bath? How do you get rid of that used up, soapy water filled with your dead skin cells (sorry, it's true...)? You WRING THAT RAG OUT!!! When you wake up in the morning, what the first thing your body usually does? Doesn't it YAWN and STRETCH?? HMMM.....

Throughout the day, take the time to stretch your body.

Don't worry if you don't realize that you ALREADY know how to do that... Your body knows which ways feel good, and it will DO IT. Now....

We've been talking about physical relaxation for the most part. Let's talk a little about mental relaxation - relaxation of the mind and spirit.

The Roman Emperor, Marcus Aurelius, had an amazing technique for mental relaxation, one that I use quiet frequently with good results:

"... Men seek retreats for themselves; Houses in the country, seashores and mountains; and thou art want to desire such things very much, but this is altogether the mark of the most common sort of men, for it is in the power whenever thou shalt choose to retire into THYSELF. For nowhere, either with more quiet or more freedom from trouble, does a man retire than into his own soul, particularly when he has within him such thoughts that by looking into them he is immediately in perfect tranquility, and I affirm that tranquility is nothing else than the good ordering of the mind. Constantly then give to thyself this RETREAT and RENEW

THYSELF..."

He was a very smart man, and taking into consideration that advances modern research has made in regards to relaxation and rejuvenation, we know now that Marcus was talking about relaxing and going to alpha brainwave, which has the characteristics and benefits mentioned earlier.

When we close our eyes, we sort of retire into ourselves. Our attention tends to become focused within. We attempt to shut out the outside world, so the only stimulus we have is our own thoughts, feelings, and memories. Have you ever closed your eyes and remembered something from long ago, only to come out of it and realize that you were lost in a memory?

It happens all the time without our conscious awareness, and what Marcus Aurelius wants us to do is to GO INSIDE and get totally absorbed in that FEELING of relaxation. In your imagination, you can recall your favorite place to relax, and you can be there. Use all of your senses to recreate the feeling of being there:

Remember what you heard

Remember what you felt

Remember what you saw

Remember what you smelled

Remember what you tasted

Another very effective- and very easy - way to elicit the relaxation response is to practice Deep breathing. Deep breathing is important because it moves the Lymph fluid throughout the lymphatic system. If you don't know already, the lymphatic system is responsible for producing lymphocytes, which are the long arms of your immune system. Lymph fluid, which is that clear fluid that you might see when you get a cut or some other wound, is only moved during activity - like walking or exercising. Deep breathing has also been proven to move the lymph fluid.

Although exercise moves the stuff, the best form of exercise to move the lymph around is REBOUNDING - which is bouncing up and down on a mini trampoline. If you have the money, then do yourself - and your family - a huge favor and get a mini trampoline. Jumping on a rebounder is a total body exercise in every sense of the word. It works using gravity, acceleration, and deceleration. At the height of the bounce, you're essentially weightless, and when you come down, which you definitely will, your mass is doubled. This effect stimulates all the muscles, cells and organs in your body. Imagine what kind of workout you'll get when you bounce on this thing for 5 minutes!!!

The stimulation caused by jumping up and down actually stimulates all the cells in your body. This means that you even get a cellular workout!!! You can find a good one at any place that sells sporting goods. There are MANY benefits that come from rebounding and you'll be thankful that you got one. Here are just some of the things to think about until you get your own rebounder:

- Reduce Stress
- Improve Circulation
- Stimulate the flow of your lymphatic system

- Help you see better

- Detoxify fatty tissue

In case you're wondering, NASA scientists make use of the rebounder when they want to get in shape quickly to endure the G forces present as they do their extra planetary affairs.

The best thing about rebounding is that it is low impact, meaning that if you have joint or back problems, you can still bounce and receive the benefits.

Back to deep breathing....

There are two types of breathing that we normally do, consciously or unconsciously. The first type is Chest Breathing. Chest breathing is relatively shallow. The chest expands and the shoulders rise as the lungs take in air. Under stress, we all have a tendency to breathe shallowly. Breathing can become irregular, involving both holding your breath and exhaling completely. Because of this pattern, your breathing may feel constricted, creating uncomfortable of not getting enough air. Breathing from the chest can cause symptoms such as shortness of breath and tightness in your chest. Our culture has taught many of us to breathe in this way exclusively.

Diaphragmatic breathing is what we want to do CONSCIOUSLY. Normally, when we are relaxed and feeling at ease with the world around us, we breathe deeply and naturally. By "deep", I mean to say that we tend to breathe long and deeply. It's like drinking your favorite drink; you want to savor it and enjoy the flavor for as long as you can, right? However, when we get stressed out, our breathing becomes shallower and we don't utilize the full amount of our lung capacity. Stress causes the Diaphragm to become stuck. For those of you who don't know, the diaphragm is a thin muscle that sits underneath the lungs. Their job is to help the lungs suck in air and help them exhale carbon dioxide. When the diaphragm is free, it can move up and down freely and do its job as it was designed to.

However...

When it becomes stuck, our breathing becomes shallower and as a result, we don't have as much energy as we should because we can't get sufficient air to turn up our metabolism.

If you take a look at a child and notice their midsection, it's not like the average adults: Ripped with muscles. Hey, the ability to tense your muscle is important, especially the muscles in the abdomen area, because they provide protection. There lies a difference in the abdomen of a child and the average adult. It's smoother and tends to stick out more. It's not fat; it's really their lungs that you're seeing. Children have amazing lung capacity and as a result, amazing energy. When you watch a child breath, you'll notice that the stomach moves in and out or up and down. Proper breathing is breathing like a healthy child. Of course, other factors play a part in how we generate energy, but our breathing plays a MAJOR role in the process.

Here's an exercise that has many benefits, including increasing circulation, and enhancing the functioning of every cell, organ, and gland:

1) Firmly place your left hand under the center of your ribcage and place your right hand on top of it. With your hands flat, pull your elbows close to your body so that you are hugging your

midsection.

2) Inhale deeply and push your body towards your hands while your hands push back against your body. Hold your breath and push hard. Although there is no set amount of time, the longer you hold your breath and push (without becoming lightheaded), the better.

3) Release your breath naturally along with your hands.

4) Repeat two more times.

Now…

Once your diaphragm is all freed up and can do its job the way it was designed to, you can start to practice deep breathing throughout the day. The proper way to breathe deeply is to breathe in through the nose and out through the mouth. Breathe in for 5 seconds, hold for 5 seconds, and release to a count of 5. Repeat until you feel your body relax. Breathe like your sniffing smoothing that smells good...and exhale as if you're fogging up a car window.

The exhale should make a "haaaaaaa" sound. You're allowing the breath to flow out; you're not "pushing" it out. Can you see the difference? Your breath will naturally flow out on its own.

This type of breathing is not only relaxing to your nervous system, but it also ensures that your body inhales the most oxygen possible... Exhaling through the mouth ensures that you exhale the most carbon dioxide possible.

If you want to make this deep breathing even more fun than it right now and engage your imagination, as you breathe in, imagine breathing in your favorite color. Can you easily bring your favorite color to mind right now as you're reading this? More interestingly, can you bring to mind a color that you dislike?

There have been some interesting findings in the field of Color Therapy and with daily experimentation; you may find your own. Essentially, each color is a form of vibration (energy) and by breathing in certain colors, you can have certain effects on your physiology. Even more interesting is the theory that all foods have certain colors in them and that by eating certain foods (colors), you can treat different diseases in the body. Here's a basic guideline of various colors and what they can do for you. Keep in mind that because you may be 'hooked up" differently than me, the colors may not have the same effect for you as they do for me/ the rest of the planet:

1) Red: stimulates; increases vitality and passion; releases adrenaline; raises body temperature. Can help mammy glands to secrete more milk.
   Red foods: beets, black cherries, blackberries, radishes, red cabbage, spinach

2) Orange – influences digestion and assimilation; builds physical energy; improves self confidence and positive thinking; used to treat spleen and kidney dysfunctions.

3) Yellow – stimulates mental faculties (helps to improve visualization ability); increases optimism, cheerfulness; used to treat skin diseases. Stimulates liver and gallbladder.

4) Green – soothing, influences blood pressure; used to treat tired nerves.

5) Blue – treats feverish conditions, bleeding, germs, nervous irritation; calms the mind; treats rheumatism. Here's an interesting fact: blue light has replaced blood transfusions

for about 30,000 babies a year in the US. However, because the blue light began to irritate the nurses on duty, many hospitals added gold lamps to soothe the staff and restore their nerves.

6) Indigo – used to treat obsessions, nervous disorders, insomnia, and diseases of the eyes, ears, and nose.

7) Violet – stimulates the nervous system, used to treat neurosis, cerebral diseases, neuralgia, rheumatism and epilepsy. Maintains potassium in the body.

8) Copper – treats bone and joint problems

9) Silver – used to treat sciatic conditions

10) Gold – restores your nerves

11) Black – Protective

12) Brown – grounds you

13) Pink – treats spleen conditions, plumps up the skin, helps with asthma

The list goes on, and this will give you a simple starting with which to notice and experiment. Do you have too much green or red in your life? Do you need more pink?

You may find that breathing is Cyan today annoys you where

as Mustard yellow is the color for today. Your body instinctively knows what's best for it, so allow it to help you see what's best for both of you. Imagine moving that color throughout your body and sense which organs/ligaments need which colors.

Better yet, can you think of your favorite song? What song is it that is so awesome that when you hear it, you automatically start to feel better? As you think about that song in your head, just relax and breathe. My personal favorite color is navy blue aka royal blue. I hate purple though ☹ What's YOUR favorite color?

If you want an extra boost, you can imagine releasing all the stress in tension in your body as you release your breath. The cool thing about breathing is that is it one of the few physiological processes that we have some control over and it happens to be the most effective one to control. When you gain control over your breathing, you can start to gain control over your feelings; it's the "gateway physiological event". Have you ever noticed the way you breathe when you're experiencing certain emotional states? For instance, have you noticed the way you breathe when you hear good news? Have you noticed the way you breathe when you're panicking or upset about something? The differences here are very important and when you start to pay attention to those differences, you can control yourself and your life and interactions will be the better for that control. Understand?

As a general rule, anything that gets you moving and breathing a little harder will energize you. Have you ever seen an energetic person sitting still? I haven't. Movement creates energy, as odd as it sounds. Have you ever noticed how when you sit still for a long time, you start to actually get sleepy? You would think that the opposite would be the case, as you're "saving" energy, right? Wrong!!!

Movement deepens your breathing, which increases your physical energy.

There's a very big difference between your body NEEDING sleep and your body FALLING ASLEEP because you're not moving around and increasing your breathing.

Remember, you control your body, not the other way around. If you want to increase your energy, then create the demand for that energy by moving around. It seems too simple to be true, but it works. Whenever I'm feeling "stuck", I get up and move around. After a few minutes, my state is much more productive and I can think much more clearly.

Now…

How does it feel to know that you now have a simple technique for resetting your nervous system so you can do what you like doing longer and better? You're welcome☺

Well...

Here's an awesome technique that takes a couple of minutes, but when you do this, you'll feel better immediately.

You're going to start to use your neurovasculars consciously. Neurovasculars are specific points in your body that when you touch and hold them, blood is distributed to that area. But something amazing starts to happen when you do that… Any organ that is associated with that specific pair of neurovasculars is fed with blood and consequently, nutrients. There are many neurovasculars in the body, the most effective ones are located on your forehead about an inch above your eyebrows. These neurovasculars, when held, will cause the blood to flow back up into your forebrain so you can think clearly.

As I mentioned earlier in this book, when you're stressed out, blood immediately leaves your forebrain and flows down into your arms and legs and prepares you to fight or flee (remember the fight or flight response?).

Without further ado…

The next time you feel hit by stress and feel overwhelmed or highly emotional:

1) Lightly place your fingertips on your forehead, covering the frontal eminences aka the "oh my god!!!" points:

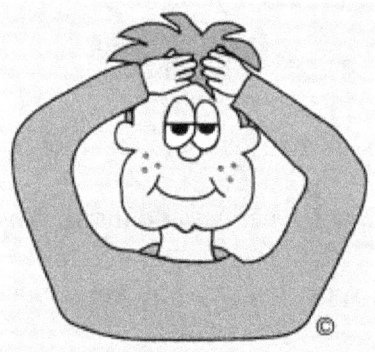

2) Put your thumbs on your temples next to your eyes, breathing deeply (in through your nose and out through your mouth)

3) As the blood returns to your forebrain over the next few minutes, you will find yourself beginning to think more clearly. It is that simple!!!

The really cool thing about this technique is that the more you do it, the more your body takes on the habit of keeping the blood in your forebrain. What does this mean for you? It means that the one little stressor that used to screw up your day no longer affects you as it did before. As a matter of fact, you will have the ability to deal with that stressor with a clear mind!!!

As you keep your fingers on those points, you'll notice a sensation under your fingertips. That's the sensation of the blood flowing back up to your forebrain.

Another way you can use this technique is to mentally rehearse how you want to act and react in a particular context. Let's say for instance that you're nervous riding public transport. However, this may be your only means of transportation at the moment and you're riding it determines your livelihood. What's a person to do?

Do this: Close your eyes and as you think about that situation that gets you all nervous and anxious, imagine yourself reacting calmly. Imagine how your body will feel when it's completely relaxed and at ease with the environment. As you keep your eyes closed and your fingertips on your "oh my god" points, imagine what you would see if you were in that environment. How do you want to react in that situation? Imagine yourself reacting in the way you want to react.

Is this awesome to know when you're getting ready to take a test?

Is this awesome to know when you're driving in rush hour traffic?

How can this be useful for you when you're preparing to get your

drivers' license?

Wait….

It Gets Better!!

You can use this technique as you're taking a test!!! As your

sitting there taking your test, cursing yourself for going to Canada

the night before when you should have been studying, you can take

your index and middle fingers, and thumb of your non writing hand

to hold your neurovasculars, so you can keep the blood in your

forebrain as your taking the test!! How awesome is that????

You can even help your friends and family members relax by

holding THEIR neurovascular points when they are stressed or

anxious or afraid. Your mother, father, brother, sister,

boyfriend/girlfriend will appreciate you even more!!!

As you getting ready to physically enter the environment that

was causing you stress and anxiety, take a moment to take a few

deep breaths and blow out all that tension and fear. In situations like these, you'll find it really easy to breathe deeply because your brain needs that oxygen to do its magic and your body needs the oxygen to regulate all those very important physiological processes… like breathing☺

Now, before you put down this book, just realize something very important here: the techniques in this book will help you relieve some the stress your under, however, keep in mind that until you get rid of the CAUSE of the stress, namely the situation and people that are causing you to feel that way and replace them with the people and situations that you DO WANT, then things will always be the same.

Once you practice these techniques and make them a part of your daily behaviors, you'll start to experience more energy and vitality.

Remember, that just reading this book won't allow you to absorb these concepts and make them a part of your life. Practice makes perfect.

YOU HAVE TO DO THE DRILLS!!!!

Can you stop right now… and think of all the places where you can use this information.

At work?

At home?

At meetings?

Anywhere you need a quick recharge is pretty much fair
game, right? That's it for now. Please, enjoy your book and read it
whenever you get a chance to do so.

For more awesome information on relaxation, visit my blog today
and subscribe!!

https://seathebiggerpicture.wordpress.com/

PART 2

How to Be Your Own Personal Trainer and

Get The Results YOU Want!!!

Disclaimer: <u>Please consult with your physician before you begin and exercise program and please consult a registered dietician before you begin a change in your diet. This manual is not intended to cure or heal anything and is not a substitute for medical treatment. If you have a medical condition, then please consult your physician to learn of proper treatments.</u>

Imagine having the motivation and the determination to start an exercise program… and stick to it easily and have fun as you do it…

What would your life be like if you could become your own Personal Trainer?

How would you feel when you can get out of bed and exercise and be full of vitality and energy?

How would you feel if you could motivate yourself and easily reach your fitness goals?

I want you to realize that you can become your own "personal trainer" and become a specimen of health and fitness. You can also teach your own family to eat healthy. And you can do it for FREE. In many ways, you are already your own personal trainer, but… if you're not reaching your fitness goals, then you're probably doing something wrong… or worse, not doing something at all. It's ok, because we can tweak a few things to get you to where you want to be.

Now, before you keep reading, I want you to perform a little experiment: I want you to look at your television. Now, as you look at the television, I want you to "think" about changing it. Don't actually get up and change it; just sit there and think about changing it. Let me know what happens… I know lots of different exercises to help you increase your strength and flexibility, but to not USE THEM, it's like you sitting there and thinking about changing your television. What skills do you have that you aren't using in your daily life?

In case you haven't yet realized what I'm getting at, my point is this: like the television, exercise will only work for you when you get up and DO IT. It does absolutely no good to sit there and KNOW all the exercises you can do; you have to create your own routine and then follow it consistently to see results. Thinking about exercise is good, and you'll discover why as you continue to read. You want to research exercise as much as possible, to let you know what your options are. Like many things, people tend to jump into things before they analyze the situation and their options. Do your research on exercise so that you can become aware of all the possibilities that are attuned to you own personality. Some people like bacon and eggs, some people like a hot fudge Sunday (I like both☺).

If you could design your own perfect exercise routine, how would you design it? What exercises would you include in your perfect workout program? What exercise would you start with? If you could sit down right now and write out your perfect exercise program, what would you write?

If there's one thing that both you and I know, it's this: we all know what areas we need to improve on and which areas we need to do away with completely, but that's something better left for another day. Start to think of yourself as a naked mannequin; if you could dress yourself in any type of clothing, what kind of clothing would you want to wear in?

Before you read the rest of this manual, there are a few things that you should know: I'm a Certified Personal Trainer and have been helping people change their lives for about 10 years now. Like most personal trainers, I decided to become certified as a personal trainer because I love fitness and I truly believe that when each person in the world takes control of their health and start to become more active, then we can be more productive and have more fun. In addition, if EVERYONE on the planet radiated health and vitality, then we'd live in a much warmer place☺

One important thing that you need to know is how you motivate yourself to get stuff done. When you stop and think about a task or project that you felt extremely motivated to complete, what comes to your mind?

What motivates you to get stuff done?

Do you talk to yourself? (Technically, we all talk to ourselves all day long with our own "internal dialogue")

Do you see big, bright pictures of your outcomes?

Are you proactive with your health, or are you reactive?

When I say "proactive" and "reactive", I mean to say: do you actively take care of your health and body or do you wait to go to the doctor and find out what's going on inside before you take care of your health? In case you haven't noticed yet, it is absolutely crucial that you start to be proactive when it comes to being healthy and fit. Don't sit and wait for your next doctors' appointment to discover whether or not you have high cholesterol.

Now...

I want to talk about Setting Goals: Setting a realistic goal is ESSENTIAL to meeting not only your exercise outcomes, but those important outcomes in other areas of your life. There are many effective models that you can use to set your own goals, and here's the one that I use to set my own goals, because it's extremely effective and very simple to remember.

The S.M.A.R.T method. "S.M.A.R.T" stands for:

- <u>Specific</u> – a defined, specific goal (I.E. I want to lose ten pounds or I want to build more defined arms) is much easier to focus on than vague statements, like "I want to get into shape". See the difference?

- <u>Measurable</u> – Define measurable, tangible goals; then it will be clear that the goal has been achieved, and thus enhance your motivation. Have a way to measure your progress. What will you see when you reach your goal? What will you be feeling? What will you be hearing? You need some sort of evidence procedure that lets you know that you've reached your outcome.

- <u>Action oriented</u> – When you choose your goals, write out details of the plan, including the days, times, duration, and how intensely you want to exercise. Have your plan in a place where you can see it all the time. Ask yourself: "If I did know what to do to get this ball rolling, then what would I know?"

- Realistic/Relevant – Choosing goals that are realistic and appropriate is critical for ensuring the success of your exercise plan; attainable goals help to set you up for success.

- Timed – a timed goal is one with a Target Date for reassessing yourself. Having a target date gives you something to work toward and gives you focus. Another good thing about having a deadline is that it automatically causes you to work to meet the deadline. Deadlines can bring intensity to any plans that we have. Deadlines help you find a source of energy inside of you that you probably aren't aware of. Deadlines create a sense of urgency deep inside of you, and when you have that feeling of urgency attached to a specific goal, your subconscious mind will definitely take notice and realize that achieving this outcome is important to and so, it is important to "it". I'm sure that you notice the difference between "something you don't really care about getting done" and "something that I know will change my life for the BETTER the SOONER I get it done".

Many powerful corporations use the SMART method for business success and growth, and now you're going to use it become healthier.

One thing I'd like to mention is the importance of setting a long term health and fitness goals. It is okay to want to lose a few pounds to fit into a dress or tuxedo for a wedding, but, crash dieting is not the way to do it. Short term goals are important, because they can be the stepping stones that build the road that will lead us to our major outcomes/long term goals. If you need to, seek out a qualified dietician in your area that can help you eat properly so that you can lose weight and have more energy.

Crash diets are a short term option, because many times when a person loses massive amounts of weight while following the weight tends to come back just as fast. It's much better to eat properly and develop a habit of being active than to crash diet. There's a difference between following a specific diet if you're going to have an operation performed on you and following that same eating plan for the long term. Not good… Start to focus on the long term. I ask myself this question all the time when I feel myself starting to slip or adopt unhealthy habits of eating, exercising, and most importantly, thinking. It's a question that I find to be very powerfully effective in building character. Remember, our brains are plastic in nature, and you have the ability to change for the better. People change all the time and you're going to change too… and the amazing thing is that YOU can control the direction in which you change. The one thing that I believe without a doubt is that change is one of the few constants, and that we can change as we wish.

Start to ask yourself:

"What type of person do I want to be when 5 years from now?"

As you sit down and allow the answers to come to your mind, you might mysteriously feel compelled to pick up a pen and some paper… and write out all the traits and habits that you want to have. If you could picture your "perfect self", how would you look? What types of things would you be doing? I find this exercise to be very centering and maybe you'll discover that you start to feel more and more centered when you start to ask yourself this question when you feel like you're "slipping". This little thought exercise is the most important in this book, and as you start to develop the habits that you want, then you'll start to see why…

Now…

Here's a simple technique that will help you start to thinking about exercise in a more positive light. This exercise works best to help you change those bad feelings and reactions to exercise into something a little better:

1) When you think about exercise, how do you feel? Now…

2) As you notice where in your body you feel that feeling

3) What would it feel like if you could take that feeling… and allow it to get smaller and weaker, to the point where it just fades away….

4) And in its place, you start to feel a feeling of POWER and STRENGTH….

5) As you start to think about all the things that you associate with strength and power…maybe you can see a picture of a lion, or maybe you can see a picture of a ferocious tiger getting ready to maul its prey….

6) And as that feeling grows stronger inside of you now…

7) You start to smile, as you realize how awesome life will be when you start to exercise more regularly…

8) And as you start to smile to yourself and feel good about exercising. You suddenly see a picture of yourself smiling… and dripping with sweat… you might even see a picture of yourself talking with your friends about exercise…. Now…

9) Have your feelings about exercise changed yet? If not, read the above steps again until you start to feel better about exercising.

If you read through the above exercise, then you might have notice how powerful an impact your Internal Representations have on your thoughts and feelings. Our internal representations can be images, sounds, feelings, smells, and even tastes. We all have a primary modality, which is basically the one sense that we prefer to receive information from the outside world and with which we code or store information in our minds. Why is important to know your own primary modality? Well, once you become aware of your primary modality, you can realize how best you can communicate with yourself and motivate yourself to get stuff done.

The five primary modalities are:

- Visual (See)

- Auditory (Hear)

- Kinesthetic (feel)

- Olfactory (Smell)

- Gustatory (taste)

The really cool thing about internal representations is that you can link together many representations and create a "thought loop". You can tie one good thought, to another good thought, to another good thought, so that when you think about each separate thought (link in the chain), you automatically think about the others. Now, I wonder how you can create a "thought loop" ™ that will cause you to automatically think about exercise in a fun and positive way….

Thought Loops© are extremely easy to create, because we as people tend to think in associations. In other words, when you think about "A", you automatically start to think about "B", and when you think about "B", you automatically start to think about "C", and so on and so on…. Why not take advantage of the way that you already think and set up a positive "Thought loop" ©.

Sometimes, we get caught up in a negative thought loop, and we continue to think about negative thoughts. Thought loops are always there… always working… in fact, we can even have thought loops attached to objects!!! When you think of some object that is precious to you and that you cherish with all of your heart? Now, as you allow that object to come to your mind naturally, notice what memories or feelings are associated with it. Are you starting to realize how common thought loops are in your daily life? If you haven't noticed yet, a Thought Loop is a chain of associations. When you create your own thought chains consciously, you'll discover how much positive impact they will have in you and on your life. You can even program yourself to think specific thoughts when you perform specific actions. Say, for instance, that you want to remember or start to run more frequently (or whatever exercise that you love to do): you can say to yourself:

"Whenever I'm (in the car/in the shower/on the couch), I'm to suddenly start thinking about jogging/doing yoga/doing tai chi/going for a hike).… If you haven't noticed yet, I place lots of importance on controlling your thoughts. Every idea starts in your head, and when you stop… and look around you now, you start to notice all the things that you use in your daily life… and you start to realize that all those thing started off as IDEAS, something that is by most definitions "not real", since we "think" we can't observe it… but I'm sure that you can look at a person and tell how they might be feeling can't you? Our thoughts are that powerful… when you realize how much control you have over your own thinking, then you'll start to feel more confident and powerful.

Now…

After working with a few clients, I realized that much of the time, having access to equipment and having the necessary time to get into better shape isn't the problem; there's some sort of psychological issue that's working beneath the surface that prevents a person from taking the necessary actions that will help them reach their fitness goals. There can be many things that can cause you to have negative associations with exercise. It's up to you to look inside yourself… and notice what associations you have when it comes to exercise. This is very important, because when you discover WHY it is you don't like to exercise, you can start to construct some HOW'S.

Another common thing that I hear from people all the time is that they just don't know where to start. Doing research on health and fitness is CRUCIAL because you have to have a program that works for you; and for you to have a program, you have to do your research and look at all the exercises that are available so that you can piece them together in a manner that's just right for your needs and physical ability. Your mind is like a blank slate, and you need to fill it everything you can concerning exercise.

Beginning an exercise program or making a change in eating habits without having the proper information is like a person that wants to go on a trip without a map; the person doesn't have a destination in mind, but they know that they want to go on a trip. Now, how far do you think they'll get, if they get anywhere?

Another reason that many people don't start or stick with an exercise program or a change in eating habits is because they don't have the proper MOTIVATION to help them reach their goals; they know that they don't want to be fat anymore, but they don't know where they want to be instead. Knowing what you DON'T WANT is only half the battle; knowing what you DO WANT is the other half of the battle. Both are equally important. This is why goal setting models like the SMART model are important for helping you to become clearer on what it is that you do want.

You need to know what you DON'T WANT so that you have reasons to push you away from your current state. You need to know what you DO WANT and you need to make it so compelling that you automatically do all the things necessary to achieve that outcome. You need to find a way to make yourself feel so bad about your current situation that you find yourself being automatically pushed away from it. You have to find a way to make it so disgusting that you can't stand to experience that condition anymore…. And you have to find something that so much better, that you find yourself automatically pulled to it, like a powerful magnet pulling a piece of steel.

That's the reason why I wrote this book; many people have the DESIRE to lose weight and get into shape, but they just don't have the knowledge and the proper motivation to do what it takes to get into shape.

The ancient Greeks prescribed exercise as medicine. The Greek physician, Galen, developed a system of medicine that treated individuals according to their specific "temperament", or personality. He prescribes specific exercises to his patients based on their personality. Although I'm not a doctor, I feel absolutely confident in saying that one of the Master Keys to staying in shape is find a form of exercise that you find to be FUN.

Some people love walking.

Some people love lifting weights.

Some people love going for hikes or canoeing.

Some people love the calming effect and increased energy flow that Tai chi has on them.

Some people enjoy the relaxed feeling they get after a yoga session.

Some people love intense spinning and cycling classes.

Some people like swinging kettle bells (I do☺)

The point is to find something that YOU enjoy.

When you think about it, doesn't that make perfect sense? It's like "retirement": I truly believe that when you absolutely love what you do, then you'd never ever think about retiring from it.

When exercise becomes fun for you, then you wouldn't even think of "retiring" from it. I LOVE Warren Buffet, because he loves what he does and he wouldn't dare consider retiring from it. When I go to the park for a run or to sprint, I'm always energized and inspired by the older people that are up there EVERY morning walking or riding their bikes, because on a deep level, they realize the importance staying healthy and they are reaping the benefits. Isn't that the type of elderly person that you want to become?

Exercise and its benefits

Ever since high school, the thought of going to gym brought a heavy case of the shivers on. The thought of exercising seemed like torture, but believe it or not, your gym teacher had your health in mind. Here are some of the benefits associated with exercise:

Health Benefits of Exercise and Physical Activity:

- ☐ Reduce the risk of premature death

- ☐ Reduce the risk of developing and/or dying from heart disease

- Reduce high blood pressure or the risk of developing high blood pressure

- Reduce high cholesterol or the risk of developing high cholesterol

- Reduce the risk of developing colon cancer and breast cancer

- Reduce the risk of developing diabetes

- Reduce or maintain body weight or body fat

- Build and maintain healthy muscles, bones, and joints

- Reduce depression and anxiety

- Improve psychological well-being

- Enhanced work, recreation, and sport performance

- Strengthen your cardiovascular and respiratory systems

- Manage your weight

Exercise and Depression

Exercise fights depression by activating the neurotransmitters — chemicals used by your nerve cells to communicate with one another — associated with avoiding depression. Those neurotransmitters are serotonin and nor epinephrine. The levels of those neurotransmitters and their balance with each other play a role in how you react to daily events. When you experience depression, the level of serotonin, norepinephrine or both may be out of sync.

Exercise may help synchronize those brain chemicals.

Exercise also stimulates the production of endorphins — other neurotransmitters that produce feelings of well-being, provide for "natural" pain relief, and help you relax. So, did you have a stressful day at work and need to blow off some steam?

A workout at the gym or a brisk 30-minute walk can help you calm down. You can turn an ordinary walk into a supercharged, calorie workout by focusing on your breathing: breath in comfortably for 5 or 6 steps, hold for a second, and breathe out at a comfortable rate. I do this all the time when I walk. I find that it acts as a kind of meditation which helps me clear my mind and also energizes my body. And best of all, It's totally free and you didn't have to wait in line at a noisy gym to get some good quality exercise!

Please keep in mind that I'm not saying that exercise is a CURE for depression, but it is definitely a nice tool in your arsenal in the battle against it. If you're depressed, please seek out professional help to discover the root cause and fix it.

Besides all of these benefits, you'll feel GREAT!! You'll have all the energy you need to go through your day and more.

My job as a trainer is to provide my clients with the necessary instruction in terms of using proper form and developing awareness of what muscles are being worked so that they can be EMPOWERED and be independent. Stop and think about it: who REALLY wants to spend $100 dollars a session when they can do the same thing in the privacy of their own home for FREE? I sure as hell wouldn't, would you?

I feel, as a personal trainer, if you're not exercising on your own after training with for a month with me AND you're not enjoying it, then I haven't fully done my job. That's just the standard to which I hold myself. Let's make it fun!!

I believe that it is my duty to help my clients develop the necessary habits that will allow them to stay in shape. If a client wants to pay for a consultation to refresh themselves on using the proper form, then that's a different matter but, I feel that being a personal trainer is about teaching a person to be self sufficient and more independent.

One thing that you as a client need to realize is that here is no such thing as "50/50". When you stop and think about what it means to give "50/50", you'll realize that this implies that each person only gives HALF of the effort that they are capable of giving. It's much more accurate to give "100/100", don't you think?

Now…

Let's talk about habits. What exactly is a habit? A habit is a behavior or action that we perform automatically. Habits are created through repetition. As an interesting side note, do you know what a monk's attire was called? A habit!!! We all have habits that we develop and we all have habits that we've had since we were little boys and girls. I'm sure you've heard the word "habitual" before, haven't you? And I'm sure you've heard the term "force of habit" before, right? Well, I believe that people are as unhealthy or as out of shape as their HABITS.

Healthy people are in the HABIT of being active and being outdoors. Out of shape people are in the habit of being sedentary and not being active. Healthy people are in the habit of eating healthy foods and consuming good fats. Unhealthy people typically consume loads of processed foods and fried foods. Now, I'm not saying that healthy people don't indulge in fried foods every now and then (I love a piece of fried chicken every now and then, and ice cream… and brownies….), and I'm not saying that an unhealthy person doesn't eat healthy every now and then. What I'm saying is that the habits that we have an indicator of how healthy or unhealthy we are. Healthy habits make for healthy people; unhealthy habits make for unhealthy people. Doesn't that just make perfect sense?

Well, here's the amazing thing about habits; you can develop new ones that will replace the old ones. It sort of like washing out a dirty cup that's got grime and grease stuck to it; as you continue to rinse out the grease and grime (your bad habits) with clean water (new, better habits), the cup becomes clean, to the point where it's like new!!!

Our brains are amazingly flexible and can easily create new neural pathways, the result of which is new habits. Neuroscientists refer to this phenomenon as "Neuro-plasticity", referring to the plastic properties of the brain. If you've ever seen melted plastic, then you know what I'm talking about. Notice how that plastic will easily mould to the new shape. Well, you don't have to melt your brain in order to develop new habits that will last for the rest of your lifetime.

Now...

Before we move on, I want to talk a little bit about self image. The way that you perceive yourself determines how you interact with the world. If you see yourself as a shy person, then you'll act shy. If you see yourself as outgoing and friendly, then you'll see yourself as such. How do you see yourself? Do you see yourself as lazy or active? If you see yourself as lazy, then you need to remember times when you've been active.

Can you remember a time when you felt really energized and productive?

Can you remember a time when you got a lot of work done and you felt good that you did?

As you remember that experience:

Remember what you saw

Remember what you heard

Remember what you felt

When that experience reaches its peak, or when you feel as though you are actually relieving the moment/experience, you're going to touch yourself in a certain spot on your body. It can be anywhere; the back of your hand, your shoulder, your forehead, etc. You can even use a "key word" that will remind you of that specific experience.

Now…

The point of the little exercise is to help you remember that you have the capability to get stuff done, and what's more, you can easily get back into that state anytime you want and you can energize yourself to start exercising regularly. All you need to do is to touch yourself in that in that certain spot and say your "key word", so that you can elicit that state of excellence. You may have to elicit the memory a few times and set the physical anchor before it "sticks" and you can easily recall that state of excellence.

It's much easier than people realize to motivate yourself to get stuff done. How do you talk to yourself or what do you see that makes you want to get things done IMMEDIATELY?

What do you think will happen when you talk to yourself in that special way when you want to exercise?

Another simple way to get started exercising regularly is called "chunking". Essentially, chunking is what you call it when you break down the specific action into all the little steps that are necessary to its achievement. So, let's say that you want to "work out".

Now, you would break that down into all the little steps necessary to make it happen.

So…

1) you get dressed to exercise

2) you decide what type of exercise you're going to do (cardio, resistance, etc)

3) you grab the necessary equipment

4) you go to the specific location

5) you start to exercise

6) You get the point by now, don't you?

Chunking works because of the attention that you're paying to the details. Not everyone wants to "work out", but everyone will at least take some of the small steps that will eventually lead to the desired outcome, which is "working out". Are you starting to see how chunking works and how you can use it to develop a habit of regular exercise... know your outcome, but focus on all the little steps that it takes to get there.... Many times, people get discouraged by the "big picture" (working out), so "chunking" is an amazing way to help you feel more empowered to get in shape.

Now...

One thing that AMAZES me is that it's so simple to get into awesome shape. It's so simple that it's FREE!!! If you don't believe me, then talk to all the people that have lost weight and CONTINUE to lose weight by putting themselves and staying on a walking program. Walking is the easiest thing that we can do to get into shape. Walking stimulates your left and right brain hemispheres, balancing their activity and allowing thinking with your entire brain. There are many other health benefits of walking.

If you need more convincing, then I'm sure you may have noticed those really buff guys working out in the playgrounds and parks. I know you've seen them, or at least heard of them.

They are the guys that are doing pull-ups on the monkey bars; they are the guys that are doing decline pushups on those little toys that are shaped like animals; they are the guys that are doing laps around the entire park or playground.

I have much respect for these people because they WANT to be in shape and they realize that you don't need an expensive gym membership to do it. Do you realize that many people in the world have gym memberships and they don't even use them? Some gyms can charge up to $250 bucks for 3 months. Sure, you get all access to the gym, but how often are you really going to go in there and use the equipment.

Here's something that you can use if you have a Gym Membership, but you don't want to cancel it just yet:

1) The next time you're in the gym, possibly when you're in the locker room getting cleaned up…

2) Stop and think about all the reasons that you like coming to the gym. Allow all those reasons to flow through your mind now, no matter how weird they may seem. It only matters that YOU know what they mean. Now…

3) Really allow all those reasons to clearly stand out in your mind. If you want to, write them down so that you have a constant reminder of the things that you enjoy about the gym. You can even make those reasons stand out big and bright in your mind. You want to focus on all the positive aspects of this place.

4) The positive aspects that you become aware are going to act as Positive associations that will be attached to the gym that you frequent. Remember how I was talking about "thought loops"? Well…

5) As you think about all those things that you love about your gym, you'll notice how they automatically link together, so that when you think about one thing that you like, you automatically think about another thing that you like. Neat, right?

Unless you're a bodybuilder or a Powerlifter, then you're most likely not going to be in there every other day. Do you really want to waste all that money on something that you're not going to be using consistently? I sure as hell don't, do you? I hope not.

I think it makes much more sense that you purchase yourself a pair of dumbbells that are challenging for your current fitness level. There are SO MANY exercises that you can do with a pair of dumbbells that is ridiculous. You can get a total body workout with a pair of dumbbells and an exercise mat: really stop and think about what that means… can you imagine how much money you'll save and how much healthier you'll get when you buy a pair of dumbbells and workout in the privacy of your own home? You don't even have to buy an exercise mat; you can find a blanket or some other padding that will provide comfort and support.

Now…

Before you even start to get into shape, you need to know and become aware of your current physical condition. You have to know where you are so that when you begin your exercise program, you'll need a baseline measure against which to measure your progress. It makes no sense to just jump right into an exercise program and not have a means to gauge your progress. For all you know, you could have reached your goal years ago and you're just not aware of it!!! You could already be living the life that you want to be living, but you don't have the sensory acuity to notice it! Wouldn't it be horrible if you were living your perfect life and you weren't aware of it? As I mentioned earlier, the SMART model of goal setting is a very effective way to help you KNOW when you have reached your goal.

You can determine your current level of fitness easily by taking yourself through a Fitness Assessment. There are a variety of them and you can use one of them or all of them to determine your current level of fitness:

- Basic fitness assessment that tests your cardiovascular capacity, muscular endurance, flexibility, posture, and takes your resting heart rate. The cardiovascular component requires you to step up and down on a 12 inch high stepper for 3 minutes. The purpose of the test is to see how quickly you recover from the exertion.

- The Rockport walking test, in which you walk a mile and notice how you feel after the walk. If you can't complete the test, then you're out of shape. The faster you complete the test, the more fit you are.

- Physical agility tests.

- Graded maximal tests that require the supervision of a trained professional. An example of this would be a "stress test" that your doctor might give you if you're 40 years old or older.

Here's the good news: the basic fitness assessment and the Rockport walking test can be done for FREE. You can do them anywhere you can find a place to walk a mile and a place where you can do pushups, partial curl ups, step up and down on a stepper for 3 minutes, and check your posture and flexibility. Once you know HOW to do them, then you can perform these test for YOURSELF. If you don't have a stepper, then you can perform the Rockport walking test to assess your cardiovascular ability. If you feel more comfortable with a personal trainer performing the assessments, then by all means find a good personal trainer and have them lead you through them.

Let's talk about what YOUR criterion for "being fit" is. What kinds of things do you want to be doing?
What kinds of things will you be doing when you're in better shape?

You need to have a "Criterial Equivalence", or evidence that lets you know that you've reached your fitness goals. When you have your criteria already in your mind, then you can determine whether or not you've reached your goal… and you can also determine what you need to do to get there. "Health" and "fitness" mean many things to many people. Some people think that you need to as big as the Incredible Hulk to be fit. Some people feel that you need to be able to run a 10k marathon every week in order to be healthy. To each his own. You have to become aware of what YOUR criteria of fitness and health is. Many people want more "endurance". Well, I know what the word "endurance" means for me and I know when I have more endurance. You have to know what "more endurance" means to YOU. Understand?

Speaking of relativity.

Keeping in mind that all things are relative, what's easy for you in terms of exercise may be a difficult undertaking for someone else, and vice versa. I tell the people that I train that you have to "start where you are at". Many people set a standard for themselves and they feel disappointed or frustrated when they don't express that standard. Or worse, many people compare themselves to others. Set your own standards and have the patience to do everything necessary to reach it and live it. Setting a standard is fine, because it will give you something to work toward. One of the keys to sticking with a weight loss or fitness program is to set a REALISTIC goal and realistic time frame. On average, you can expect to lose 2 pounds a week. Expecting to lose 10 pounds a week is not very realistic or healthy in the longer view.

Now, let's talk about "excuses". We all have them. We all have perceived obstacles that can prevent us from reaching our fitness goals. Most of us don't realize however that the very excuses that they have also contain the SOLUTION to getting around the roadblock. For instance, one excuse that I hear A LOT is "…I can't workout; it's too cold…". Well, what do you do when you're cold? Don't you put on more clothes so that you get warmer? Or maybe I'm the only human on the planet that does that… did you know that your body responds to exercise in many ways one of which is increasing your body temperature.

Hmmm……

The point I'm trying to make is that there's a solution to every problem; you just have to search for it and find it. This little bit of wisdom applies not only to exercise and fitness; you can use this knowledge to improve your life. One simple thing that you can do to become aware of all your objections is to:

1) Get a piece of paper and WRITE THEM OUT. Don't stop writing until you've listed every excuse or objection to getting in shape.

2) Once you've written out your objections, at the TOP of that sheet of paper, you're going to write the following question: "…If there was a way to get around these roadblocks, then what would that way be?". When you write this question at the top of the sheet of paper, you're going to have a constant focus on finding the SOLUTIONS to your roadblocks. The

question at the top is a reference point. Questions are very powerful ways to communicate with your subconscious mind and get solutions.

There's something that I strongly believe and I want to share it with you now: I truly believe that when an outcome is extremely important to you, there aren't enough excuses to keep you from working towards its achievement.

In other words…

Where there is the will (desire), There is a way. You may have noticed that I used the term "subconscious mind" in the above paragraph. I apologize if I assumed that everyone reading this knows about the subconscious mind and the role it plays in your daily life. If not then I'll explain:

As you may already know, we each have both a left brain hemisphere and a right brain hemisphere. Each hemisphere of our brains is designed to carry out specific functions. These hemispheres of the mind have been referred to as the "objective mind" and the "subjective mind". The left brain hemisphere (objective), for example, is the brain hemisphere that's most active in people during our day to day activities. Many scientists refer to this duality as the "bicameral mind". The left brain helps us keeps track of time and is very linear. Our left brain is also responsible for our ability to count. The right brain (subjective) deals with our creativity and our ability to imagine and visualize. In addition to having a Bicameral Mind, we have a Conscious Mind and A subconscious mind.

The conscious mind can be described as your ego, or the part of you that is CONSCIOUSLY reading this right now and as you notice the words in front of you and the shapes and the color of the white background, you can easily become aware of what your conscious mind is. Your conscious mind is the part of you that consciously makes a decision to do certain things, like get up and go get something to eat, or step on a bug on the ground beneath you. While your conscious mind seems easy enough to understand, your subconscious mind is a totally different bowl of soup. Your subconscious mind is ALWAYS alert and awake; whereas your conscious mind sorts of "blanks out" and turns back "on" when you fall asleep and when you wake up, your subconscious mind does NOT. Your subconscious mind is constantly awake as it should be, because it makes sure that you keep breathing; it makes sure that your heart keeps beating; it makes sure that you keep going no.1 and no.2. In other words, your subconscious mind is that part of which controls the involuntary functions of your body, like the ones mentioned above. In fact, many cultures have referred to the subconscious mind as "the silent witness". The only "involuntary" function that we can exert some degree of control over is our breathing. We can consciously control our breathing rate and in turn, we can control our states of being and our emotions, as well as increase our energy and our vitality. More on all these awesome things later.

You may be asking yourself "…why is all this information about my conscious and subconscious mind so important and how is this going to help me get in shape?" Well, if you remember what I just said about the subconscious mind, you'll remember that your subconscious mind is ALWAYS awake. It is always paying attention. Just because you stole that money and no one saw, your subconscious mind was paying attention and it REMEMBERS. In fact, one of the functions of your subconscious mind is that it acts as a "storage center" for your memories. In fact, your subconscious mind functions in many ways a like recorder, video and voice; any impression that you have ever experienced is in your "Storehouse" of memory right now. Anything that you have lived through was noticed AND recorded by your subconscious mind. Everything you've ever read is stored deeply in your subconscious mind, just waiting for your instruction to recall it. Think of all your senses as being "windows", through which you AND your subconscious mind experience the world around you.

Another amazing function of your subconscious mind is because it remembers how to do things; it helps you live your life much easier because it's where we store our HABITS. It remembers names, dates, places, faces, etc. IT REMEMBERS EVERYTHING. I think we've all had the experience of wanting to remember the name of a person or a location; you have that question in your mind and you keep asking yourself over and over "what the hell was the name of so-and-so?" you drop the question, and then, sometime later, maybe a few hours later or a day later, the answer suddenly pops into your head. From where did it come? I'll give you two guesses.

All the skills that you've ever learned are being carried out by subconscious mind. Think about something that you do every day, like driving or walking. Do you have to consciously place on foot in front of the other, or do you just pick a destination and the next thing you know, you're standing right there. Or when you get in your car and drive, does it always feel like your "first time", or do you automatically check your mirrors, step on the brake, turn on the car, and pull out onto the street, and head off to your destination? I really hope that each time you drive doesn't feel like it's the first time for you, because I would feel bad after I cussed you out.

When you think about something that was hard for you when you first learned to do it, and as you continued to practice and get the hang of it, it became easier and easier to the point where it's second nature. Can you think of some skill that you have right now that was hard and now it's easy? As you think about that now, I want you to realize that it's much easier now because your subconscious mind learns by REPETITION. That last bit was so important that I'm going to repeat it below this and capitalize and italicize it:

YOUR SUBSCONCIOUS MIND LEARNS BY REPETITION.

Are you allowing all of this really important information to sink into your head and really absorb this? I can tell you that this knowledge of your subconscious mind has much more far reaching applications than establishing a lifelong habit of having fun while you exercise.

Simply put, the more you practice something, the more automatic it becomes to the point where it's natural and easy to do it, and you can't even imagine what your life would be like if you DIDN'T do it. When you think of something in your life that you couldn't do without, what comes to your mind?
Now…

This huge lecture on the left/right hemispheres of the brain and the conscious and unconscious mind is important because when you realize what equipment you have to work with, you have a much easier time getting the job done. Sure, you can pick up a broken egg with a fork, but it comes up easier when you use a towel or napkin, don't you think? The reason I gave the mini "lecture" is because your subconscious mind can be your most powerful ally… or your worst enemy.

Since you're an intelligent person (you HAVE to be because you're reading this☺), I'm sure that you realize that your subconscious mind stores ALL of your habits, including your eating habits… it's okay, I know that you realized that before I stated it.

The more forms of exercise that you learn and become familiar, the more OPTIONS you have. It's almost as if you'll have access to an ENCYCLOPEDIA of exercises. I wonder how exciting exercise can be when you think of all the ways you can mix and match different type of exercise… If you've ever watched "The Matrix" with Keanu Reeves and Lawrence Fishburne, you might remember the scene after Neo was awakened from the matrix and shown the true nature of the world. One of the "operators" uploads data directly into Neo's mind/brain. He uploads many different forms of martial arts within seconds. Although you won't experience anything like that, you can take advantage of Muscle Memory. Muscle Memory or "motor memory" is just what it sounds like: your muscles have the ability to "remember" various motor movements, provided you repeat them enough. One perfect example of motor memory is…. Riding a bike!!! It's one of those things that you always remember how to do.

Our muscles and nervous system have the ability to memorize motor acts. Learning tai chi is a way to utilize muscle memory. Playing tennis is a way to utilize muscle memory. Muscle memory is utilized during weight training sessions and cardio sessions. To give you an even clearer example of muscle memory, can you remember a time when stopped working out for a long time… and then, suddenly, mysteriously, you decide to go for a run. Your muscles already "remember" how to run; it's just that you're body might not be in the shape that it used to be in when you were running regularly.

Thanks to muscle memory, you don't have to relearn how to jog. When you learn different forms of exercise, you can be like Neo, or Trinity (if you're a lady☺) and access them from your "motor database" anytime you want!!! Isn't that amazing? When you start to think of exercise in terms of developing new skills and abilities, don't you start to feel better about it? The key to memorizing motor acts is repetition!!!

There's something really amazing about the subconscious mind: it can communicate with you, but more importantly, you can communicate with it… there's a sort of two way communication. If you doubt the validity of what I'm saying, then think about your dreams. Do you realize that when you have a dream about

107

something, much of the time it's your subconscious mind trying to communicate with you through the imagery you see in your dreams? This is a common example of the subconscious mind "reaching up" and trying to get your attention.

There are many techniques that you can use to communicate with your subconscious mind. One very popular…and very powerful method is hypnosis using guided imagery. During a hypnotic session, the hypnotist will lead you into a deeply relaxed state of mind, during which they will direct you to create mental imagery (sounds, feelings, sights, etc) which serve as instructions to your subconscious mind. You see, words are fine for communicating with your subconscious mind, but the words only serve to help your conscious mind create the imagery, which is picked up by your subconscious mind. The uses of hypnosis and its effectiveness are very well documented, and range from curing many things, such as phobias (i.e. A fear of heights) to even natural breast enlargement!! If you'll remember what I said when I described all the functions of the subconscious mind, you'll remember that I mentioned that "it" controls all of those involuntary bodily functions. Now… let's put everything together:

When you relax yourself deeply, you can communicate with your subconscious mind by creating mental pictures of your desired outcome and your subconscious mind will do everything it can to make that outcome a reality.

Doesn't it seem like you always receive inspiration from God/ Your guides when you're in a deeply relaxed state?

This is the reason why I place so much emphasis on focusing on what you DO WANT: Since the subconscious mind learns best through repetition, what do you think happens when you're constantly thinking about and talking about what you DON'T WANT? This is also the reason many self improvement authors tell you to WRITE OUT YOUR GOALS. When you right them out is like filtering out a pan of rocks and gold nuggets: as you continue to shake loose more of the dirt (what you don't want), then you start to reveal more of the gold nuggets (what you do want). The act of writing things out is also a very powerful stimulus and message to your subconscious mind.

Your subconscious mind can also help you get into better shape and establish healthier habits of living when you set CUES in your external environment that cause you to think about exercise which in turn, lead to the actual physical activity that you want to do.

You see, not too many people realize how much of an impact your thoughts have over your actions. Our thoughts, even though they are not "real" or measurable, have a very real impact on our daily lives. It's like this: you don't see the wind, but you can see the effect that it has on the tree that it blows against. Our thoughts work in much the same way; you can be happy one moment and then before you know it, you're completely depressed and feeling like garbage, and you can't understand why… and it happens so fast that you aren't even consciously aware of the process. What happens is that sometimes, when you think about something that's really depressing, or when you remember a really sad event in your life, your body almost instantly goes back into the same state that you were when you were experiencing the actual event!! The same thing happens when you remember a time when you felt really strong and confident… when you remember a time when you felt like you could fly… the fact that our thoughts have a powerful influence over our bodies and our health has been proven by science many times over. The founder of Applied Kinesiology, George Goodheart, developed a technique called "muscle testing, wherein which a person's muscles are tested to determine what foods and objects actually strengthen them….. or weaken them. You can even test which rooms in your house are most compatible/incompatible with your bodies' energy. They also discovered something really amazing:

A positive thought will actually keep you strong!
Holding a negative thought will cause you to weaken!

We'll talk more about muscle testing and what happens when you hold a positive thought in your mind later on… right now, you're going to set your own external cues so that you are triggered to think about exercising and eating properly. To do this:

1) You're going to want to use some sticky notes so that you can place our "cues" all around your house and even around your work area. If possible, get some multi colored sticky pads.

2) On each sticky pad, write a little reminder of what it is you want to remember to do. For instance, if you don't drink enough water, you're going to put on a sticky pad the question: "Did you remember to drink water today?" On another sticky pad, which you're going to place somewhere in your office or wherever it is that you work from, you're going to put "have you taken the stairs yet?" On another sticky pad, which you might want to put in your car or someplace like that, you're going to write: "Have you eaten 3-5 small meals today?" Are you starting to get the point? The basic premise of this little reminder technique is that you write out what it is that you do want to do, and you put them some place where you can see them every day. It's deceptively simple, but tremendously powerful. It works by repetition. The more you see these sticky pads around, the more your subconscious mind gets the message that you should be doing what's listed on the sticky pad. Are you starting to wonder about all the places that you can place sticky pads with helpful reminders?

In addition to the "Sticky Cue", you're going to want to make a "health checklist". This health checklist is simply a list of the basic necessities that everyone needs to stay healthy. You can customize your list however you choose, but here's my own checklist that I keep on my wall.

Health Check List

1) Water

2) Fresh Air

3) Raise your heart rate 3 times a day for 30 seconds.

4) Stretch your body

5) Review my outcomes

6) List the things that I'm grateful for

7) Get up and take go for walk

8) Relax and enjoy yourself

9) Connect with friends and family

10) Do 5 things today that will help me reach my outcomes

Your own health checklist may have more or less than the one that you see above, but it doesn't matter; the purpose of your checklist is to remind you to do things that will help make your life a little better. On your own list, you might add "look a stranger in the eye and smile" or "help an elderly person today" or "take some time to meditate". The options are infinite and can be organized however you like.

How to Create your own Perfect Personal Trainer!!!!

In Neuro Linguistic Programming, there's an effective process called "modeling", in which you study and emulate the behaviors of individuals so that you can learn their skills. Practitioners of NLP have a saying that goes "anything that you can do, I can do…". We all have skills and abilities, and we all have specific steps that we take to make those skills and abilities work. The basic premise of "modeling is that when I understand the process that YOU use, I can emulate that strategy and get the same results. Cool, right?

By now, you're probably wondering: "how is modeling going to help me?" Well, when you model the behaviors of people that are already fit, you can become fit. When you think about someone in your circle of friends or family that absolutely fit and healthy, who comes to your mind?

What types of things do they eat?

What types of activities do they do?

Who can serve as good role models? Well… anybody who's already done what you want to accomplish.

Yes, I know it sounds weird, but it's very true. Just because a person may be dead and gone, doesn't mean that all the great accomplishments that they were responsible for are dead. That would mean that because Martin Luther King died, his famous speech was never heard by many of us on the planet, and his presence didn't help people become more tolerant. That would mean that all the amazing insights that Bruce Lee shared with the world in regards to martial arts are gone and buried. I guess a better way to say it is like this:

Although a person's physical body may be dead and gone, their SPIRIT is still very much alive. It's a concept that took me a long time to understand, but I am so grateful that I finally do.

By now, you see my point…. Anybody can serve as a role model.

What fitness experts can you use as YOUR role models? Amir Campbell ?!?! Richard Simmons? Tony Horton? Billy Blanks? Your Best friend? The sky is the limit…. Anyone that you can study, you can emulate.

On a much deeper level, we are all capable of doing anything that anybody else has done. We all have all have the POTENTIAL to do great things. There's the matter of living up to that potential that's a totally different matter.

There something even more amazing: you can actually "ask" these fitness experts for advice!!! And you can get answers from them. If you're starting to think that I'm nuts, then think about this: how many times have you seen those bumper stickers that read "what would Jesus do?" Well, you can adapt that simple mental process to your own fitness goals when you ask:

"What would xxx do?

I'm not exactly sure how it works, but I do know that it works partly by dissociating you from yourself and places your focus on something outside yourself that does have some answers.

If you were walking down the street and you happened to step on a $100 dollar bill, would you care more about where it came from or would care more about the fact that you FOUND THE FREAKING MONEY!!!!

You don't realize it yet, but you have an amazing ability to visualize easily. When I ask you to think about a red polar bear with a birthday hat, how quickly can you do that? We do this automatically all day, every day. We have the capacity to create amazing things in our imagination, and what's even more amazing is the fact that these mental constructs can have a powerful impact on our thinking and on the way we act.

I'm going to lead you through a process that will allow you to create your own personal trainer, a mental construct that will act as a motivator for you during your exercise programming. This mental construct is also going to act as a reminder of your fitness goals. This mental construct is going to become your symbol of health and fitness.

Before you sit down and create your "fitness symbol", you need to do a little ground work to build a foundation. The cool thing about this is that you can do it while you're wide awake. Imagine what it would be like if your perfect personal trainer were standing right in front of, about 3 feet away.

You need to:

1) Get a pen and some paper.

2) Write out every single quality that you want in a personal trainer. How do they talk? How do they stand? How muscular are they? Is your personal trainer a man or a woman? Are the kind and gentle, or are they tough and commanding? List every single trait that you would look for in your perfect personal trainer. How does your personal trainer walk? How do they talk? How do they dress? What kinds of foods do they eat? Remember, this is YOUR mental construct and you can make it act and look and anyway YOU choose. It doesn't have to make sense to anybody else; it only has to make sense to you. What you are doing here is sort of creating the "skeleton" for your construct.

3) This is the most important step of the process, I feel: You're going to give your personal trainer a NAME. If you could give them ANY name, what would you name them? The reason you want to give your construct a name is because

it allows you to "call him or her up" when you need advice or motivation.

4) You're going to want to memorize the remaining directions because you'll be leading yourself into a deeply relaxed state.

5) Once that's done, you want to find a place where you can close your eyes and relax. You're going to energize your construct so that it will help you keep on track. Please refer to one of the relaxation techniques from earlier.

6) Now, once you're feeling deeply relaxed, you're going to visualize your perfect personal trainer. As you remember all the qualities and characteristics, you're going to make a picture of them in front of you. Now... if you're having a hard time visualizing your personal trainer, just imagine that you're describing him/her to your best friend. How are describing them?

7) As you see them standing there before you, and you notice what kind of clothing they are wearing... you're going to give them instructions such as:

"You're my personal trainer and it's your job to help me reach my goals. When I call your name (mentally or whispered to yourself), you're going to show up and you're going to help me in the way that I need it…"

It doesn't have to be the exact wording, but something similar to that will do. Remember, you're talking to your subconscious mind, and when you talk to it, you want to speak to it just like you were speaking to yourself or a close friend. When you stop and think about it, you can't get any closer than a "silent witness" that's been with you your entire life and making life easier, can you?

In case you haven't noticed yet, you can use this technique to attract an ACTUAL personal trainer!!! Use your criteria to find a personal trainer that "clicks" perfectly with you. Of course, you want to research your potential trainers' track record and his/her results, because you want to know how much experience they have to offer you.

Part 3

**Quick and Easy Guide to Eating Right for Weight Loss and More**

**Energy!!!**

Before you read any further, I want you to Stop!!!... and realize

something very important… I want to really allow this to sink in

easily and naturally into your unconscious mind….

You have The Power To Choose.

It might not seem like much, but it is.

Remember this the next time you go to the supermarket and you're

thinking of good food to bring home and prepare.

You can CHOOSE to buy good food or junk food or as I like to call them "Discretionary calories..."

You can choose to work for another and make them rich OR follow your passion and make YOURSELF rich.

You can CHOOSE to get up, get out of the house, get some fresh air and start to feel better and better. Walking really is good for you, in so many ways.

You Can Choose.

Oh yeah, just one more thing before you read this manual through... and I promise you that you are going to want to read it all the way through to The Last Word, because you are going to find LOTS and LOTS of really awesome things that you can put to use today...

No matter where you are Right Now, just remember that we start where we are at, and as we Living, Breathing human beings, we are constantly growing and evolving, and even though you may have

those periods or times in your life where you feel like you're stuck...
Believe me, I've been there.

Some of you may know that feeling; it is almost as if you're walking along in huge, wide, expansive field with lots of bright yellow and red flowers.... And as you're walking along in this Massive field... You suddenly...mysteriously run into a brick wall. Try as you might, there's no way around it... there's no way over it...

What's a person to do?

I like to think of this little "roadblock" as nature's way of telling me that I need to find a new way to do things.

Use that opportunity to get your personal life in order. Get rid of things you don't need, and start looking to add more of things you really do need.

Alright. Enough of all this talk about your POWER to CHOOSE. Let's move on, shall we?

Now...

Eating to live, not the other way around

What does that mean? Eating to live means that you eat the necessary amount of food to sustain you in your daily tasks/ missions/ fun activity thingies. Essentially, since food is fuel, you want to start to view food AS fuel; it's tasty and awesome looking sometimes, but it's only there to help power us through our days/nights/overnights. It's there to help us rebuild our bodies after the long hard day it's been through. It's there to help bring families together at holidays… and then tear them apart because your nephew thinks he's stronger than you and can finally fight you for the last piece of apple pie… he *thinks*. We instinctively know this; we fall short however, when things that we don't like or can't control pop up. Sometimes is it's just a matter of listening to your body when it tells you it's reached its Full Point.

You know the feeling: you've eaten so much that your stomach feels like it's carrying around your bowling balls. Don't get me wrong; I totally understand. As human beings, our most highly develop sense is our Visual Sense. Because the eyes are the windows to our souls and even more remarkably, connected directly to our brains, we "eat first with our eyes. More specifically, a whole host of biochemical and physiological reactions begins when we see delicious food; hormones are pumped out, memories are remembered, drool is drooled. It's the reason why pancake and burger commercials are so effective: the advertisers do everything possible to make the food LOOK as tasty as possible, so tasty that after watching a certain commercial, you find yourself wanting to get up out of your comfy pants and go get some.

I've been there. Many times, we eat food, just because we're bored. How many times has this happened to you: you've been sitting there, minding your own business when all of a sudden you feel like eating, yet you're not even hungry? What's going on? They're many things that might be happening:

1) You ate food, but you didn't eat enough and your body wants more

2) You just ate food, but it didn't have the right amount of macro and micronutrients in it, so you want more.

3) Your brain may need more fuel, as it's greedy and it accounts for a good percentage of your body's air, water, and food usage.

4) You broke up with your girlfriend, so you need a gallon of Ice Cream to sooth the pain and help you fall asleep, because your comfy pants just aren't that warm

By putting food in the second place, you have more energy to accomplish your life's goals. Simple rules of eating are as follows:

1) Eat when hungry, but not starving.

2) Eat a balanced meal of fruits, veggies, and your fave source of protein.

3) Drink water to help fill your stomach and carry all those delicious nutrients to your cells to make new skin, etc

4) Back away from the table when your stomach feels 70-80% full. This is a subjective number, but you have to play around to figure out what it means to YOU.

Another great way to let yourself know that you've had enough food is to ask yourself:

"Can I go for a swim right now with this food in my belly?"

Or this question:

"Can I go workout an hour from now and not be worried about this food slowing me down? Will it be all digested and ready to be put to use by the time I get to my Geri- fit class?"

These 2 questions help to orient your thinking to focus on eating what you need for the moment. More specifically, they orient you to eating to LIVE.

We all have issues with food; some people eat with a storage mentality, some people have low appetites. We all tend to swing from one end of the spectrum to the next.

The key to changing which direction you swing is to think about the triggers that make you eat towards those extremes. Our brains are funny that way: we hear a sound, smell a smell, see a sight and it triggers a flood of memories and associations which can trigger physical actions and reactions i.e. you hear a certain song and you feel a certain way and think about a certain person.

With preemptive action and conscious effort, we can destroy those triggers and start fresh with a clean state to go forward.

If you, Like Me, love good food and love to eat it as well, then when you hear the word "diet", you feel like you're watching someone walk down the street with a delicious chocolate cupcake with white frosting and rainbow colored sprinkles on top… and then watching them drop that cupcake and seeing the cupcake the ground and become all inedible and stuff… Well that's how I feel when I hear that word? How do you feel when you hear the word "diet"? Or better yet, how do you feel when you hear the words " … you have to go on a diet…"?

Well, if I told you that you can still eat good food and lose body fat and build some muscle mass, would you want to know you can do that?
Of Course you want to learn how to do that!!!

Before we jump right in here, I'm going to share with you the most important tool that you will ever use to help you get slim and stay that way for as long as you want…
Are you ready? Here it goes…

The most important thing for you to do is <u>Be Aware.</u> Common sense, right? Well, you'd be surprised. The key to eating healthy is to be aware of what you're putting into your body. This is YOUR body. You have to take care of it because you and your body are one, from this moment on until the time when you fall asleep for the last time... Got it? Think of your body as a cute, cuddly pet that you are taking care of... for the rest of your life.

Think about it this way: Would you rather live in a house with bad insulation and terrible plumbing, plumbing that backs up every single day…
or…
Would you rather live in a home with AWESOME plumbing and awesome insulation?

The easiest way to start to eat healthier is to Be Curious. Be curious about food. Be curious about the nutrients…or lack thereof in the foods you like. I think you'll be surprised when you research your favorite foods and *Become Aware* of its nutritional profile… if it has one. There's one website that I would recommend to people to get them started in the right direction to eating properly and healthy.

http://www.whfoods.com/

Just type in the food that you want to know about and you'll learn all about its nutritional profile: Here's the website:

I discovered this website years ago and I am so thankful that I did because it has been indispensible in helping me to eat healthy and helping my clients and it has an added benefit: when you know that you are eating food that is healthy, you start to feel good inside…. You feel good inside because you know that you putting really stuff into your body…

Now, speaking of Nutrient Density…

This is a fancy term for eating food that has a lot of nutrients in it. That's it. Nutrient dense foods have lots of nutrients and are usually low in calories, so they pack a double benefit. Here are some examples of nutrient dense foods:

- Strawberries

- Pomegranate juice

- Blackberries

- Plums

- Raspberries

- Blueberries

- Papaya

- Brazil Nuts

- Oranges

- Tofu

- Beans (all varieties)

  Flaxseed,

- Sunflower Seeds

This list is by no means exhaustive. The website that I provided with a few pages back (http://www.whfoods.com) is an excellent resource for choosing nutrient dense foods. You owe it to yourself – and your family – to go check out this website and learn more about the awesome health benefits of some seemingly "simple" foods.

Another common mistake that people make when attempting to lose weight is that they starve themselves. This is not good. You need to eat at 3-5 small meals a day, as opposed to eating 2 or 3 big meals through the day. There's a big difference here: when you eat

When you eat 2-3 huge meals a day, your body often doesn't have enough energy because of a clogging effect, sort of like pouring too much water down a drain at once; it gets to the point where the draining process slows down. In this context however, it means that we tend to store more fat. Many people resort to ineffective snacking techniques (I.e. grabbing everything in sight), which works for awhile, but then you find that you're hungrier and hungrier. This is one of the reasons that many people actually GAIN weight when they go on a diet!!! With 3-5 small meals through the day, you provide your body with a steady supply of energy.

Make sure that each meal contains protein, carbs, and some form of good fat. Each meal must be a complete meal in terms of nutrients. If you need help with this, then consult a nutritionist in your area. There are many that you can find when you look in your local yellow pages.

WE ALL GO TO THE FRIDGE!!!

So… on a huge sheet of paper, in big letters… you're going to write:

Are You Reaching For…

- Fruit/Veggie

- Lean Meat/Eggs

- Nuts

- Water

This works beautifully because of the simple fact that you will see every time you go to the fridge!! Every time you see that note on the fridge, you're going to automatically think about getting something nutritious won't you?

A simple way to stop unhealthy food cravings!!!

This is something that we all go through from time to time: there's one food that we KNOW is fattening to all hell, but for some reason, you find yourself craving it intensely… to the point where you feel as though just have to have it, no matter how bad it is for, or how many laps on the treadmill that you'll have to do to burn off all those excess calories.

Now, don't get me wrong, so called "junk food" is okay to eat from time to time, and diet is NOT the only indicator of good health. In fact, there's a man who lives in England name Buster Martin. He's 104 years old – and he drinks a pint and smokes a cigarette every day. Yes, you read that right – EVERYDAY. What's even more amazing is the fact that he just ran a marathon last year. So, maybe being excessive about our diet isn't exactly the only key to health. Stress plays a major in disease, as many diseases are stress related.

Now, here's a simple way to help you take the edge of that little craving that may be standing between you and that dress that you've been dying to get back into. I'm not going to tell how it works, but I will say that it works and it works INSTANTLY:

1) Think about the food that you really like, but you know that you shouldn't be eating. On a scale of 1 to 10, how powerful are your cravings for that food? Really see that food clearly. Imagine that a plate of it is sitting in front of you and you're getting ready to eat it. Now…

   When you can see that food clearly….

2) Think about the nastiest pile of garbage that you've ever smelled in your life. Now, as you think about a huge smelly pile of garbage with loads of flies buzzing around it so loud

that you can hear them buzzing, notice how you AUTOMATICALLY start to think about "forbidden food"... Now...

3) On a scale of 1 to 10, how powerful is your craving for that food? If that craving didn't decrease, then as you think about that food, think about a food that you absolutely HATE. As you think about that food that you absolutely hate, notice how you automatically start to think about that food that you're compulsively drawn to eat.

What would it be like if that food that you eat compulsively were to suddenly grow smaller and smaller in size until it just...disappears into nothingness. What would it be like if that food that you eat compulsively were to suddenly and mysteriously change from color to completely black and white. How compelled do you feel to it?

If the above technique didn't work amazingly well, then try reasoning with your subconscious mind: tell yourself that eating this food is keeping you from being healthy and feeling amazing. The subconscious mind listens to REASON, but you have to reason with it. It won't draw logical conclusions unless you reason with it.

I realize that my writing style maybe a bit…different, and that's fine. My only intention is that you understand the principles and techniques in this manual and that you use them to help yourself become more fit and healthy. Don't you think that's fair?

As I always say: "What's the point in owning a red corvette if you're not going to drive it?" Do you think that makes sense? I want you to think of this manual as a shiny new corvette that you're going to drive it as far as it will take you.

Now let's start you on the road to energy and vitality, shall we?

One question that I get a lot from people that want to start an exercise regimen and want to know what to eat to promote energy and endurance is "what's _something healthy that I can eat for/lunch/breakfast/dinner?"_
Well…

As a general rule of thumb (I don't know what that means and why a thumb would have a rule designated to it…) you want to choose Lean protein, good fats, and ***complex carbohydrate for lasting energy and to prevent you from "crashing".*** I'm sure you know the FEELING of crashing. If you don't know, then let me describe it accurately as I can at 9am in the morning:

You're humming along just fine. You're walking and you're feeling fine. You're putting out work at a steady pace and all of a sudden…. Your energy levels TUMBLE and CRASH to the ground, like a kid riding a bike for the first time…

Does that FEELING SOUND familiar?

Now, you may be wondering to yourself:

What are some good examples of complex carbohydrates?

Well…

Wheat bread is a very popular and commonly known source of complex carbohydrates. You may have heard the saying," the whiter the bread, the quicker you're dead"… Well, I don't totally agree with that statement because it's kind of harsh, don't you think?

Sure, white bread is a simple carbohydrate, meaning that it is broken down quickly to simple sugars which your body uses for energy. If your only source of carbohydrates is White bread, then you might have a problem on your hands. Remember this: every food is good or bad DEPENDING ON THE CONTEXT IN WHICH IT IS EATEN.

In other words, there's a time when you can actually use the quick energy provided by simple sugars, like during a marathon race or any other activity where you are working for more than 60 minutes (however, in an endurance event, you want to get a mix of protein and carbs, as protein helps your body to make more myoglobin, which will help carry more oxygen to your cells).

However, I'm a firm believer in the bit of wisdom, "All things in moderation…". I interpret this to mean that you can have so called "bad things" in small amounts. I'll be the first to admit that some days I can't get my day started right without my tangy cranberry filled muffin… things just don't "gel" for me. I'm like those guys from those gel insert commercials… only meaner…You know how that is, don't you?

So if you enjoy white bread, just know that it's okay if you eat it here and there. Believe me, I love my pizza just like the next person (how can you be human and not like pizza?) However, if you want long lasting energy, then you're going to want give wheat bread or multigrain bread a try. There are many premade pizzas on the market that have multigrain crusts and lean protein in them. Or… you can learn to make your own healthy pizza loaded with veggies and all the toppings that YOU want!!! When you do that, you can feel confident knowing that you are eating something that's extremely healthy and you won't have the guilt feeling of "damn, I really wish I didn't eat that…".

Complex carbohydrates are broken down at a slower rate and transformed into sugar more slowly, so your body receives a steady supply of sugar to give you the energy you need to do the things you do day in and day out.

The Glycemic Index is one of the best things to happen to help people become more aware of the impact of certain foods on their energy levels and ultimately, our health: The **glycemic index**, **glycemic index**, or **GI** is a measure of the effects of carbohydrates on blood sugar levels. Carbohydrates that break down quickly during digestion and release glucose rapidly into the bloodstream have a high GI; carbohydrates that break down more slowly, releasing glucose more gradually into the bloodstream, have a low GI.

The concept was developed by Dr. David J. Jenkins and colleagues in 1980–1981 at the University of Toronto in their research to find out which foods were best for people with diabetes…"

Some good sources of complex carbohydrates are:

- Brown Rice

- Multigrain bread

- Wheat Bread

- Beans

- Green leaf lettuce (The iceberg stuff is just water and vitamin K while the Greenleaf lettuce has calcium, b vitamins, and other phytochemicals in addition to Fiber that promote health and good elimination."

The only exception to the simple carbohydrate rule is fruit. Fruits are awesome. They are packed with fiber, water and tons of vitamins and minerals, natures little energy bombs. When all else fails and you're not sure what to do, just remember this:

<u>Get Fruity!</u>

Let's talk about protein. Protein is awesome, but it's mainly for maintenance. Many people are of the belief that increasing protein intake will automatically cause you to lose weight and gain muscle. That's only partially true.

Did you know that your muscles are composed of 70 percent… WATER?!?!?!? Yes, it's true!!!

People on high protein diets lose weight because their body is using a large percentage of PROTEIN for energy. This is alright in the short term, but probably not sustainable in the long term.

Protein is not designed to be used for energy, except for times of need. Athletes who compete in endurance competitions like distance running or 10k marathons are more likely to use protein for energy to meet the demands of their sports than a person that doesn't exercise frequently or more than an hour.

Carbohydrates and Fat are primarily for energy usage. That's why we store fat: in case of emergency, our body will use that fat to keep up going. Fat is a very "inert" form of tissue, which is why it's perfect for STORAGE.

In fact, fat is so important to living that our body has the ability to convert excess carbohydrates and protein into FAT. Yes, that's how important fat is to the proper functioning of our bodies. Guess what else your body can convert into fat if there's too much of it consumed at one time....PROTEIN!!!!

Aside from its functions of providing the building blocks for healthy hair, skin, and, nails, maintaining muscle AND building new muscle (provided you've broken down the muscles with proper exercise...), protein also contributes to a feeling of fullness. Why is that the case? Well, most protein has saturated fat in it, and fat takes longer for your stomach to break it down and use it. As it stays in your stomach longer, it keeps you feeling fuller.

Protein, which is begins being digested in your stomach (carbohydrate digestion starts in your mouth), takes longer to digest and therefore provides that same feeling of fullness that fat does. Awesome!!!

Now let's talk about protein in the context of "what the hell do I eat for muscle maintenance and repair?"

Well... rule of thumb (there's that phrase again...) is to eat lean pieces of protein, where the fat has been partially or totally trimmed from it. A perfect example of this is a lean cut of steak. I'm pretty sure you seen a niece, lean piece of New York Strip steak or a nice, pink chicken breast before, haven't you? Well, those are two examples of lean pieces of protein.

When you're eating out, remember to choose lean pieces of beef or chicken or the correct amounts of your desire form of protein. Here are some more examples of lean protein:

- Cottage cheese (It's not meat or poultry, but it is protein, and it is delicious☺

- Eggs (these are a very excellent source of protein that you're body will easily absorb)

- Turkey

- Yogurt/Greek Yogurt (look for yogurt with 8 grams of sugar or less, as most yogurts have a lot tons of sugar to make them taste appetizing.. sugar sure can make almost anything taste awesome, I guess…)

- Salmon, Tuna Fish, etc

There's one thing here that I want you to be aware of before you keep reading: Eating fish like salmon and tuna fish have an added benefit in addition to the protein they provide:

Fish contains what are called Essential Fatty Acids, which are "good fats". They are called "essential" because we have to get them from the food we eat, as our body doesn't produce them on its own. These good fats have a lot of benefits associated with their consumption (that's fancy talk for "Eating"…):

- Reduce inflammation throughout your body

- Keep your blood from clotting excessively

- Maintain the fluidity of your cell membranes

- Lower the amount of lipids (fats such as cholesterol and triglycerides) circulating in the bloodstream

- Decrease platelet aggregation (sticking together),

  - Preventing excessive blood clotting

- Help prevent cancer cell growth

So, now that you're aware of fish and the omega fatty acids they contain, you realize that fish is a powerful one two punch for energy and health promotion!!!

Now, you may be wondering to yourself:

"What's a good serving size of protein to eat?

Well, when choosing your protein portions, you want to choose a piece of meat that's 3 ounces in weight – or for a better picture, a piece of meat that about the size of your palm. That's all the protein you need to fill you up and meet your maintenance and repair needs.

For the last stop on the protein express….

Protein Powders and Bars.

These are actually really good source of protein. Most of the protein powders and bars out on the market today have sources of protein that are easily absorbed by the human body, which is a good thing. The one downside that I hear a lot about protein powders and shakes is… The taste.

Some protein powders and shakes have a not so flattering taste to them… and an even not so flattering after taste. So, the manufacturers of those not so tasty bars and powders came up with a brilliant solution: Pour some sugar on it dammit!!!!

Yes, they cover up the taste…or lack thereof with sugar. This good for your taste buds, but not so good if you're watching your calories and weight. High sugar intake causes your body to release high amounts of insulin, which causes your body to store fat more easily. Not only that, but high insulin levels in your bloodstream inhibits the release of Fat Burning Hormone. So, a word to the wise:

If you're going to buy protein powders and bars, then look for a bar with very low sugar content. Some bars use sugar alcohols to get that sweet taste, and these sugar alcohols can have a …unpleasant effect on your elimination system. In other words, you might get diarrhea. You'll have to experiment with the various bars out there and see which ones are "booty friendly"… and not so booty friendly. Many artificial sugars are not absorbed by your intestines, so they just pass through, and in the process, they cause watery stools aka diarrhea. Fun!!

The same thing that applies to protein shakes applies to the protein bar: An entire protein bar may be too much, and too much of anything gets stored up as fat. Many of the protein bars on the market are as big as bricks, so it's best to eat a half of one, or even less, depending on your hunger in the moment.

Another word of caution on protein bars and powders: they are not intended to replace real food. In other words, it's not safe to completely forego food and use protein supplements. Not healthy at all. If you miss a meal and you need some protein, then have a bar or a protein shake. As a matter of fact, if you're in a rush each morning and don't have time to whip up a nice breakfast, a protein shake will do just fine. When you add the protein powder to unsweetened juice and add fruit, you'll make yourself a very delicious and nutritious protein shake that will keep you full until you can find some real, warm food!!

Just remember what I said about your body turning any excess into fat when you're making your shake: The protein you purchase may recommend 1 complete scoop as a serving, but that may be too much for your body to absorb at one time, so you can use half a scoop.

One last thing about choosing a healthy, well balanced, nutrient dense meal… You want to make sure that your meal consists of Protein, Carbohydrates, and fat. Eating a well balanced meal like this will keep you full and supply you with a steady stream of energy for hours.

Now…

Let's talk Nutritional Labels, shall we?

They are there for a reason: for you to Read and See the ingredients in the food you're eating. They are so helpful that people have clamored and requested that they be put on your favorite fast foods. Now, you can look at that burger, notice how much fat is in it, and decide whether or not that burger will help you get to where you want to go. You can look at that burger and ask yourself:

… Is eating this burger going to help me reach my weight goals?".
If the answer is no, then you're going to ask yourself a more empowering question:

"What other kind of lean protein can I eat?" You want a large variety of options so that you have more choice and power over your eating habits and ultimately, your life.

For those of you who have not seen a Nutritional Label, here's what they look like:

Nutrition Facts

Serving Size 1 cup (228g)
Servings per Container 2

Amount Per Serving

Calories 280   Calories from Fat 120

	% Daily Value*
Total Fat 13g	20%
Saturated Fat 5g	25%
Trans Fat 2g	
Cholesterol 2mg	10%
Sodium 660mg	28%
Total Carbohydrate 31g	10%
Dietary Fiber 3g	0%
Sugars 5g	
Protein 5g	

Vitamin A 4%	•	Vitamin C 2%
Calcium 15%	•	Iron 4%

*Percent Daily Values are based on a 2,000-calorie diet. Your daily values may be higher or lower depending on your calorie needs.

	Calories:	2,000	2,500
Total Fat	Less than	65g	80g
Sat Fat	Less than	20g	25g
Cholesterol	Less than	300mg	300mg
Sodium	Less than	2,400mg	2,400mg
Total Carbohydrate		300g	375g
Fiber		25g	30g

Calories per gram:
Fat 9   •   Carbohydrate 4   •   Protein 4

Just study the label above and you'll discover how they work. In a nutshell, a nutrition label lets you know what you are putting into your body when you're buying food. As a general rule, ingredients are listed from Most to Least. In other words, if you're buying milk, you'll notice that "milk" is the first ingredient listed, because it makes up the majority of the food. Then you'll notice if the milk has been fortified or not with Vitamin D (or any other nutrient it might be fortified with, depending on the type of milk it is). Simple enough, right?

Again, the main purpose of the nutrition label is to inform you of what YOU are putting into your body. You can actually look at the ingredients and fat content and ask yourself:

"Is this going to help me get to where I want to be?"

Look, we're all grownups here (unless your parents made you train with me….hehe) and I'm not here to judge you or tell you what to eat and what not to eat. All I can do is make you aware of what is healthy and what is not and leave it up to you.

One last word about moderation: My belief is that life is to be enjoyed, and that we shouldn't deny ourselves of things, because denial calls for willpower, and willpower doesn't work too well over long periods of time. Sure, you might be able to deny those cravings during the day, but what happens at night when you lower your defenses? The hunger for that food that you "shouldn't" eat comes rushing back, stronger than when it first came. You have to install positive habits in yourself through self hypnosis and constant repetition. You'll learn how to do that as you keep reading…

If there's a certain food that you want to eliminate from your diet, then I can suggest a couple of things:

1) Reduce the amount of that food gradually. Don't just quit it cold turkey. That's very hard. And not cool ☺ if you're drinking or eating two cups of xxx, then try eating one cup of xxx for a week. At the end of that week, reward yourself with some prize maybe a shopping spree? You choose the reward. Your subconscious mind thrives on pleasure and shrinks when there's the threat or potential of pain.

When you reward yourself, your subconscious mind picks up the hint that this is something that it must do more of to get rewarded. It's what you do with a dog that you're training, isn't it? When the dog sits when you command it to, don't you give it a little treat? It's all about positive reinforcement. And when you do something that you know that you shouldn't be doing, then don't curse yourself. Instead, gently remind yourself of what it is that you do want.

2) Do your research and discover the nutritional profile of the food. Once you are aware of "what's in it"… and "what's NOT in it", then you'll have an easier deciding whether or not you want to overindulge in it.

3) Get support from friends and family who also want to lose weight and eat healthier. I'm sure that there are friends and family that have the same issue and when you team up and support each other, you can help each other reduce that overindulgence of said food.

4) Tell people of your commitment to eliminate or reduce that food. When you commit to others, you can be sure that they

will remind you of your goal when they notice you slipping "off the wagon".

5) Think about the long term consequences of eating that "guilty pleasure" daily and consistently. Sure, you satisfy your craving in the short term, but in the long term, you'll have to work even harder to burn off those excess calories.

6) Thoroughly research this food and see how it's manufactured. Chances are that you will never want to eat it again.

7) Schedule in a cheat day!! If you've been sticking to your eating plan all week and you have a craving for your favorite food, then enjoy it on the weekend. It will help to reduce the energy behind the cravings by satisfying them, allowing you to continue on your journey to your desired body unhindered.

Now let's talk about 'Portion Control". We all know that we should partake of specific portions of food to ensure that we maintain a healthy weight, but many people are confused as to what those portion sizes are. You might have heard that you only need a "handful of nuts", but what do you do when you have huge freaking hands!!! And who the hell can eat JUST a handful of

nuts!!!!?!!?!? Well…

I'm going to help eliminate some of that confusion you may be

feeling about portion sizes. Below is a chart that helps you visualize

what portion sizes you need to maintain a healthy weight, courtesy

of WebMD:

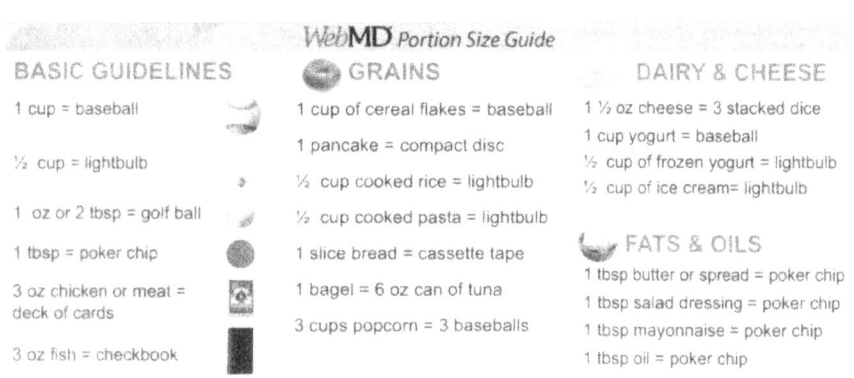

*Web**MD** Portion Size Guide*

BASIC GUIDELINES

1 cup = baseball

½ cup = lightbulb

1 oz or 2 tbsp = golf ball

1 tbsp = poker chip

3 oz chicken or meat = deck of cards

3 oz fish = checkbook

GRAINS

1 cup of cereal flakes = baseball

1 pancake = compact disc

½ cup cooked rice = lightbulb

½ cup cooked pasta = lightbulb

1 slice bread = cassette tape

1 bagel = 6 oz can of tuna

3 cups popcorn = 3 baseballs

DAIRY & CHEESE

1 ½ oz cheese = 3 stacked dice

1 cup yogurt = baseball

½ cup of frozen yogurt = lightbulb

½ cup of ice cream= lightbulb

FATS & OILS

1 tbsp butter or spread = poker chip

1 tbsp salad dressing = poker chip

1 tbsp mayonnaise = poker chip

1 tbsp oil = poker chip

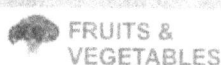 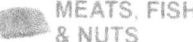

WebMD *Portion Size Guide*

FRUITS & VEGETABLES	MEATS, FISH & NUTS	MIXED DISHES
1 medium fruit = baseball	3 oz lean meat = deck of cards	1 hamburger (without bun) = deck of cards
½ cup grapes = about 16 grapes	3 oz fish = checkbook	1 cup fries = about 10 fries
1 cup strawberries = about 12 berries	3 oz tofu = deck of cards	4 oz nachos = about 7 chips
1 cup of salad greens = baseball	2 tbsp peanut butter = golf ball	3 oz meatloaf = deck of cards
1 cup carrots = about 12 baby carrots	2 tbsp hummus = golf ball	1 cup chili = basball
1 cup cooked vegetables = baseball	¼ cup almonds = 12 almonds	1 sub sandwich = about 6 inches
1 baked potato = computer mouse	¼ cup pistachios = 24 pistachios	1 burrito = about 6 inches

You can just print out this chart and put it up somewhere where you can see it and so that you can know what portion sizes are healthy.

You need to realize that your unconscious mind plays a major part in your daily life, include the things you like and dislike. This includes foods that you eat that aren't too good for you. It may not be the best for you, but you LIKE it. Do you know why you "like it"? Part of the reason is because you've probably been eating that specific food for years and you most likely have fond associations with it. It's like going to the grocery store and picking up your favorite cereal: Keep in mind that there is another company that makes the SAME EXACT

156

CEREAL. The only reason that you choose your Favorite Brand and not the "other guy's" brand is because you have many childhood associations to that particular box....

Yes. I said BOX. Your favorite cereal is no different from the cereal underneath that is sold for a LOWER price. The only reason you like this particular cereal is because of the BOX!!! The good feelings you get from eating the cereal are partially from all the sugary goodness, and now you associate that sugary goodness with that one brand of cereal. I have my favorite cereals, cereals that I've been eating since childhood. It's the same thing with peanut butter and jelly. Sure, there are a million other companies that make the EXACT SAME PEANUT BUTTER, but why is it that you choose that specific peanut butter? Well... you've most likely been eating it all your life and you've got certain associations attached to it. You can thank your Subconscious mind for that.

Your unconscious mind is that part of you that learns and remembers. Here's a perfect example: If you're a driver, Like Me, you had to learn how to do it step by step. You had to learn how to reverse. You had to learn how to parallel park. You had to learn how to control the pressure on the gas pedal so that you didn't speed up when you really wanted to slow down... you get the picture. You had to do all that stuff CONSCIOUSLY, but now, after you've been driving for some time now, you can drive easily. Your body knows what to do, when to do it. You have your unconscious mind to thank for that. Your unconscious mind is also in charge of your memory. It's a storehouse of memory, and when you request a memory, it usually can provide the information instantly. We go through what is called a Transderivational Search, during which time our subconscious mind retrieves the information we need. This transderivational search is not only a search function; it's a creation function, meaning that when you ask yourself positive questions, you get positive answers.

Can you remember a time when you saw someone's face... and try as you might, you couldn't remember their name if your life depended on it? However, maybe later that day/night, suddenly, mysteriously, that name INSTANTLY pops into your head? Again, the thanks go to your Unconscious mind. Another really cool thing about your unconscious mind is the fact that it takes care of your breathing and controls your heartbeat, your digestion, elimination, etc. (although breathing is involuntary normally, we can take control of the breathing process and in turn control your emotions. Yoga devotes much time and study to the control of breathing. If you're interested in that kind of thing then, do some research on it and see what you come up with…)

Now, here's the really amazing thing about Your Unconscious, mind. It only knows how to succeed!!! That all it knows how to do!!!

Hear me out for a moment. We have in our unconscious minds what is called a "creative mechanism". What this means is that your unconscious mind will give you exactly what you want… or don't want. Confused yet? That's good, because it means that you're thinking. It means that you actually following what I was saying.

Our unconscious minds are always alert and paying attention to everything that is going on around us. Right now it can hear things that we can't consciously hear. It records every impression that comes to us from our five senses. It remembers what you did that morning 10 years ago… it remembers everything you've ever seen and heard, and smelled…. Many cultures refer to the subconscious mind as The Silent Witness,

Our unconscious minds don't hear negatives. Words like "don't" or "can't" or "won't" get ignored by the unconscious mind, so a self suggestion such as this:

"I won't get nervous… I won't get nervous…"

Sounds like this to the unconscious mind:

"I'll get Nervous… I'll get Nervous…"

Does that sound like a suggestion that a rational person would give themselves? People all over the world are doing this…All day, Every Day!!! Unknowingly sending themselves negative messages.

This is what is meant when they say that the unconscious mind gives you what you ask for. So, are you ready to learn how to speak to your unconscious mind in the right way so that you get exactly what you want?

Okay them, listen up…

You have to speak to yourself in POSITIVE TERMS, meaning that your self-suggestion has to be focused on what you DO want. Yes, you ABSOLUTELY MUST be aware of the situation as it is at the moment. For example:

1) The situation as it is. I.e. " I have a headache"

2) The fact that you don't want to have a headache "I don't want to have a headache…"

3) The desired solution/suggestion: "…I want my head to feel fine and feel better than before."

If you don't want to be nervous… you want to be relaxed and alert and feeling good through your entire performance… or whatever the context may be. So, a proper self suggestion sounds like this:

"I won't be nervous. I'm going to relax, be alert, and when I see xxx, I'm going to smile and take deep breath…"

See the difference between giving effective suggestions to yourself and giving yourself lousy instructions that will give you more of what you DON'T want? The steps above allow you to switch your focus from PROBLEMS to SOLUTIONS. You can reach your goals easier when you make it a habit to switch from a Problem Frame to an Outcome Frame.

The easiest way to give your self-suggestions is to relax your physical body. It seems as though your subconscious mind "hears" you better when you're physically and mentally relaxed. The ancient Hawaiian people realized the importance of relaxation before you can communicate with your subconscious mind. They believed that the conscious mind carried a "charge", which is generated during the course of our day by thinking and other mental tasks. They discovered that when you relax your body completely, you can relax that "mental charge" generated by the day's activities and thus open up the lines of communication between your conscious mind and your unconscious mind. There are many ways to achieve physical and mental relaxation effortlessly. Advertisers are masters of this process and base their campaigns on the workings of the unconscious mind. Think about what happens when you're watching television: You're sitting on your couch, physically relaxed. Your mind is BORED or in other words, relaxed. Commercial after Commercial is passing in front of your eyes. Each commercial is designed to arouse in you a certain state of mind or a feeling. You might see the same commercial many times with the space of an hour. It's not like that advertiser know anything about REPETITION and the fact that your subconscious tends to follow commands that it hears OVER and OVER. Or do they?

I think we all know what happens when we see a commercial where there's a big, juicy…cheeseburger on the screen…. With crisp, green lettuce… and rich, juicy red tomatoes… with a juicy quarter pound of "pure" beef… Yummmy….
What happens when you see that commercial 10 times in the space of an hour? If you weren't thinking about a cheeseburger before you sure as hell are right now!!!
But before you even close your eyes… and relax completely… you're going to:

1) Find a sheet of paper

2) Get a pen

3) Write out the instructions you want to give yourself.

4) What types of things will you be doing when you've reached your goal? Use your imagination and act as if you've already reached your fitness goal. What kinds of thing are you doing? Are you running? Are you wearing a thong or some other skimpy underwear? Is your stomach flat?? What are you thinking? How are you feeling? How are you moving? This is called "Future Pacing", and you future pace to make sure that the desired outcome is what you want to achieve. It's like literally stepping in the future outcome and "trying it on", so to speak. Spend a little time each day "living in the future". Do you like the new conditions?

Writing out your instructions/suggestions is simple way to get them Superglued into your mind. It also serves as a powerfully stimulus to your unconscious mind, which is… stimulated by actions☺ The act of writing out your instructions is your way of letting your unconscious mind KNOW that you mean business… and this is its cue to do everything it can to help you accomplish that goal. You see, when your instructions are just "thoughts" floating around in your head,

That doesn't impress your unconscious mind that much. Writing out your instructions however, is like…

Bopping your unconscious upside the head and telling it exactly what you want!!! The act of writing something out also helps you to really focus in on what you want. There's something…magical about writing out your goals and desires.

When you write out your Self Suggestions, you're going to write them AS IF they are reality. In other words, you're going to write out your suggestion in the present tense. For example, if you want to lose some body fat and build some muscle, you're going to write out the desired weight AS IF you've already achieved that goal. When you write it out, it's going to look like this:

"I weigh a slim and healthy xxx pounds…"

To be more specific: "I keep my body fat at a manageable 12% easily"

Now, I can hear you saying: "…Amir, that's complete B.S!!! I don't weigh that right now!!! I weigh much more!!! I'm a Whale!!!" That may be true, and by the way, thinking of yourself as a whale is not the best way to lose weight. If you constantly state OUT LOUD or THINK TO YOURSELF:

"I'm a whale… I'm a whale… I'm fat…", then your Silent Witness will reinforce that image for you. You're going to eat "like a whale". Awesome, right? That's not a productive way to think of your identity, is it? What we are doing here is installing new beliefs that will cause you to automatically start to act and think in ways that will help you reach your fitness goals. And the really cool thing is this: It doesn't matter if it's true or not; the only thing that matters is that if it works or not!!!

Your conscious mind knows without a doubt that you do not YET weigh your desired weight, and we want to go directly to your subconscious mind and give it new "instructions". In time, your subconscious mind will accept the new suggestion and mold your actions to match that suggestion. Remember, your body is constantly in the process of changing, even as you're sitting there reading this.

You now have the power and the CHOICE to direct the way in which you change. You can get fatter or you can grow leaner. The choice is YOURS...

Now for the relaxation bit...

An easy way to do that is to shake your arms and legs as if you're shaking off water from them. If you want to, perform some stretches to help loosen up those tense muscles. Then, find a nice comfy chair to sit in. The reason you want to SIT UP is because our bodies are programmed to fall asleep when we're lying down. Lying down and falling asleep is a response that's been conditioned over your ENTIRE LIFETIME, no matter how many years you've been alive. That programming is as old as you are... unless you practice some form of meditation, you're going to fall asleep whenever you lay down.

Thomas Edison trained himself to relax deeply without falling asleep by holding an iron ball in one hand. When the hand holding the iron ball would drop, he would immediately wake up. Cool, right?

It's better if you sit up, in a slightly reclined position. Relaxation is key because it's easier for our unconscious minds to listen to us when we are completely relaxed. The reasons aren't important now… As you're sitting there, remember a time when you FELT really relaxed.

Once you're feeling deeply relaxed, both mentally and physically, you're going to say your instructions to yourself 5 times. You can say them out loud, or if that's not convenient, then you can say them to yourself mentally, inside your mind… And when I say out loud, I don't mean that you have to shout; you can say them to yourself in a whisper or a calm, quiet voice. Remember, we're only talking to ourselves here.

Your unconscious mind is a stickler for repetition. When you say something once, it doesn't pay too much attention, however… when you say something twice, it starts to pay closer attention, now…. When you repeat something more than three times…your unconscious NOW starts to really pay attention and it understands that this is very important. We learn by repetition. Just like the example I gave you in regards to driving.

Now, are you starting to realize how bad habits are formed in the first place?

Once you feel physically relaxed, feeling fine, you're going to relax your mind. You can relax your mind as you sit there, and visualize some peaceful scene, someplace that you've seen or been to and you found it to be really relaxing.

So here's the process:

1) Physically relax your entire body. Act as if your arms and your legs are lifeless and they do not belong to you, so you can't possibly move them. Now, if that doesn't work, then experiment and find your own ways to relax your body and your muscles.

2) Mentally relax by recalling peaceful scenes.

3) Once you feel physically and mentally relaxed, you're going to give yourself the suggestions that you wrote out before you slipped into your deeply relaxed state

I realize that, Like Me, you might be extremely busy… so busy in fact that you can hardly find time to eat (not good), let alone find a place to relax deeply and completely. So, I got something very special for you. I call it "The lazy bastard's guide to reaching your fitness goals!!!" Cool name, right? Well, I know you're not lazy. You're awesome because you're reading this!

Let me explain: I call it the "lazy bastard" method because you can get THAT MUCH closer to your nutrition and fitness goals as you lay in bed!!!

Here's how it works: Each morning, as you're waking up from that deep refreshing sleep, or that night of tossing and turning (in which case you probably didn't sleep that well), your unconscious mind is in a very receptive state and you can give yourself suggestions now!!! Your mind is producing more ALPHA brainwaves, which are associated with…. SELF HYPNOSIS!!!

This same state of relaxation occurs when you're lying in bed getting ready to fall asleep at night. Your brain is "cooling down" from the days' work, sort of like a hot engine that slowly cools down from all the work it's been doing. Your brainwaves are slowing down now…. All you have to do is write out your suggestions and repeat those to your Self a few times (remember what I said about repetition being the key to effective creation of new habits?).

This is the main reason why it's important that you focus on some goal or desire that you want to realize. During this time, your mind is very receptive and what do you think happens if THE LAST THING on your mind is the argument you had with your lover… or all the things you hate about your job?

Do you realize that your mind goes down into alpha about 15-20 minutes after you lay down in bed to fall asleep? Keep in mind that your brain cycles through the various brainwaves as you're deeply asleep. In effect, the last thing on your mind before you fall asleep is a SUGGESTION. The last state of mind that you're in before you fall asleep is what you carry with you throughout the night and what you wake up with before you head off to work… WOW!!!!

This is the main reason that I make it a RITUAL to relax and laugh before I fall asleep. Because I understand how my subconscious mind works, I realize that the best thing I can do for myself if get into a good state before I fall asleep. I watch funny movies. I write goals and outcomes. I reflect on the good things that happened to me throughout the day.

Make it your sacred duty to relax and unwind before you go to sleep and clear your head of all the stuff that you've dealt with throughout the day. Laugh before you go to sleep. Your life will thank you… You need to realize that the mood that you fall asleep in sets the "tone" for your night. Your goal is to radiate positive energy as you shut your eyes at night. If you have a mate, this is doubly important.

I like this method so much because I believe in working smart, not working hard...Like I said before, it takes us about 21-31 days to establish new habits, so to help you along, you're going to want to remember to give your self the suggestions:

1) Each Morning as your laying in bed

2) Each night as you're lying in bed, after you've changed your state to one of fun and relaxation.

Now…

Let's talk about elimination… No, not that type of "elimination" … although I'm fairly confident there are few things that you definitely can live without….

Elimination is a very important function that many of us take for granted… and it's also a Major Key to losing weight and increasing your energy. In other words, frequent pooping is important because it helps our bodies to release all those things that are no longer needed. That includes food that can't be absorbed and utilized… That even includes cells that are no longer useful to the proper functioning of our bodies.

I never used to pay too much attention to that little fact, until I was watching Eddie Murphy's "Delirious". They were taping him while he was in his dressing room getting ready to go out and perform and he was back there joking around and making everyone laugh out loud, and he said something, which was meant to be a joke, but I feel like he was actually sharing his own philosophy with this one simple statement in an old man's voice:

"The key to Longevity is havin' good eliminations!!…"

If you're not "going to the bathroom' like you're supposed to, then you might want to notice how much water you drink and what types of foods you're eating. Sometimes, when you're not able to poo, your body will hold on to that poo, and suck the water from, because it's probably not getting water from your mouth, where it's supposed to get it.

Another problem may be the lack of fiber in your diet. Fiber is filling, so it helps keep you fuller longer, and in addition, much of the material in fiber is indigestible, and this property causes your digestive system to get a "workout" in an attempt to digest the indigestible material. As a result, your large intestine is stimulated and as a result, so is your elimination.

Another reason that you might not be going poo is because of a lack of exercise. Did you know that exercise triggers, peristalsis, which the wave like motion that causes the intestines to move, and thus stimulate digestion AND elimination.

Finally....

I want to leave you with something. I want you to read these next words and allow your mind to easily absorb them... and carry them with you wherever you go... Because they will serve you well:

We are all human. We all make mistakes. We veer from the path we've chosen time and again, and the most important thing is that when you notice you've veered off track... when you notice that you're moving way off the path…you have a choice…. That's the cool thing about being a thinking being… You can:

A) Keep going in the direction that you're going and move

farther and farther from your intended destination….

Or….

B) You can open your eyes… look around you… and you can

get back on the path… and you can head towards your target.

Always have a direction in which you want to move, otherwise you're like that stagnant pool of water that doesn't move… it just gets mucky and accumulates all kinds of crap. Be like the river that is ever flowing and ever moving. You might get there quickly. It might take a little longer than you expected… But when you go around those roadblocks as you keep your goal in mind…Just know….that you will get there.

There's a saying that I'm very fond of and it's helped me in my life up to this point: There's no such things as failure… there is only feedback. You try something and if that doesn't work, you find another way and you try that…. Until you get what you want.

The best Advice I can give to you is to Keep Your Goal in View.

See it

Hear it

Feel it

Taste it

Eliminate as much as possible anything that will stop you from reaching your goal. Surround yourself with those people and things that will help reach your goal. Remember, nature abhors (hates) a vacuum, and when you create a hole…. You have to fill it with something else… or the same old stuff with rush right back in its place. Fill that hole with positivity.

Becoming consciously ware of the foods you're putting into your body is a habit that you're going to develop. Scientific research has proven that it takes us about 31 days, and constant repetition

176

to completely install a new habit into our nervous systems... But here's the really awesome thing about the Plasticity of your Brain. All it takes is once. And all though the first time is usually the most difficult when you do something. It gets easier and easier to the point where it's second nature!!!

I don't know how easily you can imagine a time in the future now.... We're you're slim and trim, and you look down at your stomach and you see that it's flat... and you start to feel good inside.... And as you look in the mirror and see the perfect body that you've always wanted... You'll look back on this moment Right Now....and you'll feel so grateful...because you kept going after what you wanted.

If you want to take a different approach, think about the law of attraction. The law of attraction states that the thoughts we constantly think create the experiences we have. What thoughts are constantly on your mind? What worries are constantly on your mind? What can you do so that those worries are now your greatest sources of joy? How can you change things around so that your life is the way that YOU want it to be?

Money and health

We all know that money is important to our survival; if you don't pay the electric bill, you and your family sleep in your cold, dark living room snuggling together tightly to generate heat. If you don't have an adequate supply of money, you can't fully provide enjoyment for your friends and family. Money is important; even more important is to use it wisely. It's not just what you earn, it's what you keep and invest.

My belief on the connection between money and health is this: when you create enough FUN streams of income, you decrease how much time spent worrying about money and spend more time enjoying your life and finding your purpose(s).

God created each one of us in unique ways. You're totally unique and there will never be another person on earth exactly like you, and it's been like that since humans being showed up on Earth. Being as unique as you are, you have the unique potential to create ways of help society prosper that have never been created before. This is where having adequate money comes into play: with more money, you buy more free time to pursue those missions.

Don't get excited; I'm not going to share some secret formula for making all the money you "need" or "want", but I will say this: The more value you create, the more money will attract. Go the extra mile in ALL your projects and you'll reap the benefits. What's it mean to go the extra mile? To me, it means that I constantly ask myself this question when working on projects: "How else can I help?"

This simple question keep you heart centered and compassionate, and you'll be amazed at the flood of ideas that will come to you when you do this. The more you give, the more you receive.

Another aspect of money that took me quite a while to understand is the fact that it's just another form of energy. Think of money like electricity; it has to go somewhere. The problem is that we (me included) can send this energy into places where it just disappears, never to be seen again. Sometimes we buy things that make us feel good for a short time and regret it later.

Wouldn't it be better if you took your extra money and put it to work for you so that it grows (pretty slowly at these interest rates, but grows nonetheless) and helps you to achieve those outcomes you want to experience? You want that beach house? Create value and save for it.

You want that Harley Davidson limited edition Golden Eagle 2020 custom ride (I made that up)? Create Value and save for it. You want that college graduation for your kids? Create Value and save for it.

I know that money is a complex issue with many people, but for me it's simple: You either have money or you don't have it, you either spend money or you save it. It's as simple as that. I also know that many people have a hard time saving money and they don't know where to start. Well, one very simple way that you can save money is by reducing all unnecessary expenditures in your budget. By "unnecessary", I mean anything that won't add long term value to your current lifestyle. Let's take for example coffee. Coffee seems like a necessity these days, in our fast paced western culture. Many people don't mind paying the cost for drinking it. The average cost of coffee is around $2.50 per cup these days, and that's for a small coffee. Imagine how much money people spend each year!!

I'm sure you heard the stories about the guy who saves up all of his change from the day, and at the end of the year, when he goes to cash in the change, he discovers that he's saved hundreds of dollars – in "small" change!!! Stop and ask yourself: "What is it that I really need!!!" Let's say that a person buys 1 cup of coffee a day at a price of 2.50. This adds up to 75 dollars per month.

Wait, there's more: If you multiply 75 dollars times 12 months, you get a figure of 900.00 dollars!!! That's $900.00 dollars a year on coffee!! Could that 900.00 be placed into your yacht/college fund?

If you really want to freak yourself out, then multiply that figure by any number of years. Keep in mind that these figures are conservative, in that I took into consideration the fact that there might actually be one person on earth who hast the discipline to say no to coffee☺

Now, we see the problem, and here are a couple of solutions:

I know how hard it is to give up something that you love, something that makes you feel good, and it's even more difficult to give it up cold turkey. So, what do you do? Replace one substance with another. Also, keep in mind the reason that most people drink coffee: To energize themselves. Well, in this book, you'll learn a few ways to energize yourself without the need for coffee. If you need to drink something to energize yourself, then consider drinking green tea. Green tea has caffeine in it as well, but just not as much. 1 cup of coffee has at least 200mg of caffeine in it, while a cup of green tea has about 50 milligrams of caffeine. All that extra caffeine is unnecessary.

Use all that money that would have been spent on coffee to buy something worthwhile. Get a jar and label it "Gift fund". It is essentially a gift after all, in two ways: One being that you use that money on something that you want. The second one being that you're not drinking all that caffeine anymore, so you won't have those nasty jitters usually associated with caffeine.

Place the money that would have been spent on coffee in that jar and watch how the amount gradually increases. I'm not saying that you have to save that money. If you need some spare change or you just want to tip the pizza guy a little bit, then you can reach into the jar and tip away.

If you're a coffee drinker and want to cut back and save money, here's how you can do it easily: You can gradually ease yourself off until one day you realize that you no longer crave coffee.

If need more reasons to drink green tea, then take a look at a few of the benefits:

CUT YOUR CANCER RISK

Several polyphenols - the potent antioxidants green tea's famous for - seem to help keep cancer cells from gaining a foothold in the body, by discouraging their growth and then squelching the creation of new blood vessels that tumors need to thrive. Study after study has found that people who regularly drink green tea reduce their risk of breast, stomach, esophagus, colon, and/or prostate cancer.

Help with weight loss

Several scientific studies have shown that green tea has ingredients in it which boost your metabolism, which can aid you in losing unwanted weight.

The most important benefit, I feel, is the antioxidants contained in green tea. Epigallocatechin gallate (EGCG), an antioxidant found in green tea, is at least 100 more times more effective than vitamin C and 25 times more effective than vitamin E at protecting cells and DNA from damage believed to be linked to cancer, heart disease and other serious illnesses. This antioxidant has twice the benefits of resveratrol, found in red wine.

Another very simple way that you can save money is by shopping for store brands. I know you might be fond of a certain brand of almond butter or a certain crème filled cookie, but let me let you in a little secret: The almonds that you find in your favorite brand are the exact same almonds found in store brands!!! The only difference is the label. So remember, when you buy that brand that you've been eating since you were a kid, you're only paying for the label and the good feelings that you associate with eating that brand.

How do I know this: Well, there was a time when I wanted to be a wealthy and powerful business man, so I majored in business administration. I don't remember much of it honestly, but what do remember, what I loved, was learning about the psychology of buying.

One thing that stuck out to me was the fact that the word "sale" is a sort of trigger. When people hear the word, they instantly think that they are getting a bargain. Most of the time, this isn't true at all. In fact, many studies and investigations have been performed, and the results were incredible: In most cases, when an item was advertised as being on "Sale", the price was in fact increased many times over the original price!!! WOW!!! Just something to think about the next time you want to spend 5 dollars on "brand xxxx" when "brand yyy" is the EXACT SAME THING at a lower cost.

Another simple thing you can do to save money is to by the Sunday paper and start clipping coupons. The savings per year are enormous when you add then up. Believe it or not, the wealthiest people in the world live quite frugally and know how to spend money wisely. I suggest that you begin to do the same and start looking for bargains. Don't be afraid that you're sacrificing quality for price. You aren't.

Of course these days there are tons of apps for saving money. There are apps for general coupons but also each individual retailer may have an app. You can often time double up on savings using a coupon and store promotion. It is worthwhile to sign up for email alerts too. They often give you something free on your birthday or advertize promotions that aren't posted anywhere else.

If you can take just one of these tips, one of these lifestyle changes, and use them to make your life the way you want it to be, then I think my job is done. I want you to carry this book with you every where if necessary, and read it whenever you have a few moments of "free time". Too often, people complain of being bored because they have nothing to do. Or so they think. "Being bored" simply means that you have time available to apply your attention and focus to some other goal or project.

You should utilize every spare moment that you have to yourself, because it's using these that we form the future that you really want to experience. Whenever you find that you're "bored", look for a sheet paper and write down a list of the things that you need in your life. You can place a maximum of five things on the list, for convenience sake. Your first item should be something that you feel that you need right now, that you can go out and buy right now if you have the money to do so.

When you've completed your list and you're sure that what you have there is what you need, then write down all the ways in which each will improve your life. Believe me, as simple as this may seem, it's an overlooked part of goal setting.

Writing down you goals does a few things:

1) It sends a signal to your subconscious mind that you really need these things, as you've created a list and therefore provided your subconscious mind with a stimulus in the form of a list, something tangible.

2) When you list the ways in which you'll benefit or not, then you allow yourself to really see whether or not this desired thing is good for you. Writing is such a simple skill, yet so many of us take it for granted or fail to realize the power you have to organize your

thoughts just by writing them down on a sheet of paper. Neat, huh?

Another way to apply yourself to something that you enjoy is to reduce the amount of time per week you watch television. Yes, I know that in this modern world we occupy, television is important to keep us up to date with current events. I realize that we MUST know the whereabouts of Paris Hilton or whom Britney Spears is running down with her car now.

If you watch television 5 hours a day, that equals to 35 hours a week spent in front of the television. That totals to 1,960 hours per year that was spent watching television. If you were to figure your salary into this equation you'd realize how much money you lost that year by watching television. You can use that time to increase your income and productivity immensely. Can you imagine how else you can put all that time to good use? I'm pretty sure you can think of a few ways even right now as you read this.

Instead of watching television so frequently, you can do other things with your time and energy. You can make "to do" lists, filled with things that you absolutely must get done in order to make your life easier and better.

I used to be a television junkie. I would spend hours in front of the television, getting lost in TV land, and then at the end of the day, I would feel regret for wasting so much time, time that I could have used to get some very important things done.

Now, whenever I have spare time, I apply the energy that I would have applied to sitting on the couch watching television to writing down ideas that can be applied to my life as it is right now. Then, when I'm sure that I've done everything that I need to do, I'll exercise a bit. I find that when I do this, I get much done in the space of one day, which might have taken me a week or more.

I truly believe that life is determined by where we place our focus. If you focus your attention on what is going inside the television, then how can you possibly focus on what's going on in your own life? This mind is indivisible and can only properly focus on one thing at a time. Why not place your focus and therefore, your energy, on something that will benefit you, something that will bring a constructive change into your life? You have to make sure that every decision that you make will benefit you, your family and your body and spirit.

Let me clarify something before we move on to the rest of this book: I have nothing against television, even though it might seem as though I do. I believe that your intentions for doing something determine how you benefit from it. If your intention for watching television is to expand your mind and then learn something new, then you'll be benefiting your mind and spirit. If you have no intention other than just to vegetate, then you won't benefit much.

I truly believe that our intentions and motives for doing things influence us and the people around us on a deeper level of being. Have you ever been sitting quietly, totally absorbed in what you're doing, when all of a sudden, something compels you to turn around. Upon turning around, you lock eyes with a complete stranger, a stranger whose been staring at you? I believe we influence each other more than you can even imagine.

So if you want to watch television, make sure that you have a positive intention for doing so. As a matter of fact, try to ensure to best of your ability that everything you do will have a positive intention and outcome for both yourself and any others that may be involved. At first, it may be a challenge to think like this, but when you see how much your life will improve because of it, I guarantee it that you will be hooked and you'll wonder how you even got along this far without this type of thinking.

Procrastination is a habit that can be easily overcome. Think of procrastination as "I'm taking my time on this project that can help my family financially and help the world…" makes you want to hurry up and get it done now, doesn't it?

Another simple way that you can increase your brainpower and potentially earning power is to carry a book to work with you. Not a novel, but a book written by author in a field of interest that you really enjoy learning about. Bring a book that you can really jump into as you eat your lunch. I frequently carry books to work, as I crave knowledge and I love learning. Let's say that the average lunch break is an hour. You bring a book to work and you read it during your lunch break while eat your organic fruits and vegetables.

You might even write down some points that you find useful and practical. Over the course of the year, this amounts to 1,680 hours of reading time. Imagine if all the knowledge that you learned in that time was put into practical application. How much more richer would you be right now? Really stop and think about the ways you can better make use of your time. Time can be money, if you want it to be.

Whenever I can find a free moment for myself, I spend my time reading books about things that interest me, things that I can apply to make my life even better than it right now. I've learned so many skills, simply because I take one hour a day to focus on something I really find interesting. The key to developing this habit to find something that you find INTERESTING. No matter what your reasons may be for being interested in it, all that's important is that you have a reason. That reason is the motivator. We all do things for a specific reason, whether we are consciously aware of that reason or not. It's far better to become of aware of the reason of which we do things, because it allows you to have more control over yourself and where you direct your energies.

One very awesome thing that I learned years ago is that it takes just as much effort to do something as it does to do something else. Let me repeat that:
IT TAKES JUST AS MUCH EFFORT TO ONE THING AS IT DOES TO DO SOMETHING ELSE!!!

One simple thing I do to get myself motivated is to promise myself a reward. I make sure that the reward is something I need in my life, something that will have great value, something that will increase my effectiveness. When all of my tasks are completed, I head out and go shopping for my reward. It's deceptively simple, but it works amazingly well because psychologists have proven that the subconscious mind has the personality of a five year old child. It responds to positive reinforcement more effectively than it does negative reinforcement.

It takes just as much energy to give up as it does to keep going and pushing to achieve your goals. It takes as much energy to stay in your house on a Friday night alone as it does to get up, take a shower, get dressed, and go out on the town and enjoy yourself. It takes as much energy to sit in front of the television and lose your mind as it does to get up right now, get a pen and paper, and write some goals that you would like to achieve. The only difference is the experiences you have as a result of the choice you make.

Let me share a story with you: a few years ago, I found myself in a situation in which it was necessary for me to leave the comfort of my warm, comfy, house and take myself to the ATM to get some money for the next day. Well, the winters in Upstate New York can be nasty, and the weather tends to drop dramatically between 10 pm and 2am. Let's just say that it's unbearably cold. Well, let me just say that I take my advice and I walk almost everywhere, much to the chagrin of friends and family. This night my walk would be made extremely slippery and dangerous, and snow had just fallen over the ice that had been on the ground for weeks.

Needless to say, I was on my butt 4 times before I made it off of my block. Honestly, I was quite discouraged. I love walking and when I don't have the space or necessary cooperation of the earth below me to walk freely, I get upset, to put it mildly; the thought occurred to me to turn back and get the money tomorrow. Then I realized that if I were to turn back, I wouldn't have my money and I couldn't do the things that I had planned to do the very next day. I needed that money to complete my scheduled tasks. I would have been set back considerably. So you know what I did? I kept going. I took my time and made sure that my vision was focused ahead of me about 7 feet, but with my vision focused on the ground before me so that I could see the telltale lump that lets you know that there's a massive lump of ice waiting to cause you all types of headaches, like a broken leg.

Every time I slipped and almost ate the snow, I remembered how much I needed that money and how important it was for me to complete the tasks that I had scheduled for myself.
I left my house at approximately 12:15am and I got back in at 3:30am. Although I was frostbitten in many places, I was happy because I got the money and I completed all of the tasks on my schedule the next day. I also learned allot about myself. I learned that at times, I can be very impatient and walking over all that ice forced me to slow down and be in the present moment.

So just remember, whenever you're faced with something that you don't want to do, remember how you will benefit from its completion.

I know firsthand that there are things that we don't want to do, but are ABSOLUTELY ESSENTIAL, so we have to do them. Why not actually feel good about doing them? Why not focus on the outcome of things that we do? Story time!

I have a friend who has some rather undesirable living conditions at the moment. He wants to move out and find a place that's all his own. He has the means to do so, as he recently got hired for a local rent to own company and is making excellent money as a driver. We talk frequently and he is constantly focusing on the negative aspects of his job, things that he doesn't really enjoy doing but are part of the job description. I think we all have jobs like that☹ Anyway, since he's a very good friend and a very hard worker, every time he mentions a negative aspect of his work, I take upon myself to ask him:

"WHAT'S SOMETHING THAT YOU REALLY ENJOY ABOUT THIS JOB?"

Without fail, he can mention at least 3 or four different aspects that he really enjoys each and every conversation we have. What I do is I have him focus on all the things that he really dislikes and I have him describe them each in detail. I have him tell how mad or bad they make him feel, which he does.

Am I trying to ruin his day? No, I want him to focus completely on all the things that he hates so that he has something to actually move away from.

Then I make it a priority to remind him of his desired outcome as a result of taking this position:

His goal to move into someplace that's all his own. A place where he can totally relax and do whatever it is he pleases. A place where he can actually hear himself think. He's thankful more and more each conversation.

We are creatures that are motivated by pleasure. In other words, we tend to move away from things that cause us pain, and we tend to move towards things that will give us pleasure, whatever they maybe.

How many days have you woken up and all though you slept through the ENTIRE night, you just feel though you could sleep another 9 hours?

This lack of desire to get up in the morning has nothing to do with your physical body, but the thoughts that you have towards the day. That's right, something so "insubstantial" as a thought has the power to render your entire body weak and unwilling.

OUR THOUGHTS AND EXPECTATIONS DETERMINE THE AMOUNT OF LIFE WE HAVE FLOWING THROUGH US. OUR THOUGHTS CAN HELP US ACHIEVE GREATNESS OR THEY CAN STOP US FROM LIVING THE LIFE THAT WE TRULY WANT TO LIVE, NOT LIVE THE LIFE THAT COMES TO US.

It's so simple, and many people realize this subconsciously. If you doubt the validity of this statement, which will soon change, read the following exercise and then attempt it. Give it your full attention and follow the instructions exactly:

Relax your body. Now imagine that your hand is really light, so light that it can float in the air with the greatest of ease. As you focus on your hand, it becomes lighter and lighter, light to the point that it wants to float to the ceiling. As you feel this lightness, just allow it to overcome your hand completely. Totally let go and allow your hand to FLOAT to the ceiling. Imagine your hand is so light and free that it is easily affected by any air current that might be present. Your hand is a leaf floating on the wind. Allow this sensation to flow through your entire body. As you sit there completely relaxed, your entire body begins to grow lighter and lighter. Your arms and legs begin to grow so light that they want to float to the ceiling. Allow your hands to do so. Allow the sensation of lightness and FREEDOM to expand to your stomach area. Completely let go and relax. You can remain in this state as long as you feel the need to do so.

Do you see how our imagination can influence our body and how we can use our imagination for better health and energy? In a nutshell, when we expect the worst to occur during a future activity (i.e. work), our body will respond in turn by creating negative emotions and negative associations (read: negative energy) with that activity.

Just the THOUGHT of the activity caused your body to grow weak. This is proof that our bodies do not know the difference between an actual "experience" and an imagined one. I know for a fact that this has happened to me many times in my life. There have been events that I have not wanted to attend, because I imagined that they might be a certain way, when in fact, upon arriving to the function, it was NOTHING like what I imagined it to be.

Can this be changed? Yes, but gradually. It takes a firm commitment and a WILLINGNESS to actually put the method into action, not a mere wishing to do so or finding excuses. So here is a exercise that you can do to help identify any feelings that you might have which are draining your precious energy and preventing you from having the health that your creator had in mind - the ability to run all day and crave more of it, the ability to make love, the lust for life that children have.

This requires some work on your part, so get a piece of paper and a pen ready. Draw a line down the middle of the paper. Write "negative" on one side and "positive" on the other.

Make a list of all the things in your life that you don't like. For instance, if you have negative characteristic traits that adversely affect your life daily life (i.e. shyness) and then write them down on a sheet of paper.

Be as thorough and concise as is possible. Leave no stone unturned, look deep into yourself and think of times in your life where a specific negative trait has kept you from getting what you desire. These go into the "negative" side of the chart.

Now, let me make a distinction here: When I use the term "negative" in relation to personality traits/habits, I use in the sense of the specific trait being detrimental to your life. Anything that affects your daily life in a negative way and prevents you from feeling good is what I term "negative"

Do the same for the side marked "positive". Write down all of your positive personality traits and the things that you desire.

Now, focus on the trait that is most detrimental to your daily life. I want you to imagine the opposite of that trait. For instance, if you're shy, imagine yourself to be an outgoing person, imagine yourself easily and NATURALLY sparking up conversations with complete strangers. Imagine what it would be like if you could look at a total stranger, notice something that you really like about them, and then compliment them on it. Imagine the sparkle in their eyes as they beam and glow because you demonstrated that you were different from the 99.9% of people on earth who are focused on themselves.

If you are "lazy" (I prefer to call it "waiting for the next big idea to hit me" :), be determined to finish a certain thing/ project on time. Set a deadline for yourself. Use the S.M.A.R.T. Goals template. Your mind is the master of your body, so it will easily obey your commands. Just have intent to do what it is you set out to do. What kind of things does the outgoing person do? Do you know anybody who's naturally outgoing and friendly? How do they act?

When I feel laziness or low motivation states creeping in, I set strict time constraints on myself and the projects I need to complete. For instance, if I'm writing an e-book, I'll set a goal to complete a certain number of useful, instantly useable pages in a certain amount of days/hours i.e. "I want to complete 20 pages of good information in the next 4 hours."

After my goal is set and the time constraint is in place, I set to work. Setting goals in this way builds intensity and it's a signal to your subconscious mind that you really do mean business and that it should do everything in its power to help you achieve your goals. Your productivity will skyrocket at rates that you would never believe in a million years.

You'll have so much free time on your hands that can be devoted to other pursuits and projects, projects that you might have always wanted to work on but couldn't because of a lack of time. When you set a goal and a time period in which you want to accomplish it, you really get things done.

If you want to learn from the master of setting goals and achieving your goals faster than you can even imagine, research Brian Tracy, or better yet, go to his website here at::

HTTP://WWW.BRIANTRACY.COM

Once you have that desired trait pinned own in your mind, I want you to spend some time focusing on that idea. You can do it anytime you have a free moment. Imagine what you would be doing if you had those desired traits. You can even list these things on a piece of paper. I find that when you write things down, they tend to go from just wispy, non-existent ideas to concrete goals that you can work to achieve.

Believe it or not, I have used this technique to overcome shyness that I had since high school. I imagined myself just walking up to strangers and talking about what was going on at the moment, and from there, whole conversations would erupt. I've even made quite a few friends in this manner. This exercise works, but only when you are DETERMINED to change. Something really helped was to change my thinking concerning so called "Strangers": I reframed a stranger into "someone that I know nothing about because I haven't spoken to them..."

Think about it: Even the very best friends that you have right now were strangers to you at some point, and you to them. Take the thought a bit further: isn't a stranger just a person whom we don't know yet that happens to radiate "Strange-ness"?

I want you to spend at least ten minutes each night before going to bed imagining the positive opposites of your negative personality. Keep at this for about 1 month FULL month and I promise that you will see changes. You must be PERSISENT. Imagine what it would be like if you had these traits. How would you act? What would you say and do if you had these traits right now? Act as if. Walk around your home rehearsing your new habits.

Listen to any feelings or thoughts that you receive, because these are messages from your subconscious mind telling you how it feels about what you are imaging. Generally, whenever I have a bad feeling about something, that's a signal that I would do better with something different. I always follow my gut and it always works out for the best. Your subconscious mind, believe it or not, knows your likes and dislikes better than you do.

Have you ever taken a course of action and then later regretted, having looked back and remembered the bad feeling that you got about it?

For instance, let's say that you wrote down "a new apartment". I want you to fully associate, or immerse yourself into the sensation of being in your new place. Imagine what it feels like to walk around uninhibited, without having to worry about bumping into anyone. How does your new place look? How big is the bathroom? Is there a couch? What do you feel in your body when you sit down on it and completely relax into it? Any windows? Where's your cooler/refrigerator? How big is it? What types of food do you have in it? How many lights do you have in your place? How much space is there? Is there enough space to do somersaults? If so, imagining doing one with enough room left over to easily do three more. What sounds can you hear from your new place? Are you in the country, the city, or on the beach?

Your list can be as long and short as you wish it to be. Continue to do this with each item on your "wish list". Incorporate feeling, hearing, and seeing. Imagine the pictures of your place to be as bright as possible. It's easier when you focus in one sense a time: For instance, when you can bring the image up anytime, then you can go ahead and focus on the sensations that you would feel AS IF you were there right now. Remember, it's your imagination, so you have full control. You can make every mental image as bright or as dim as you so please. You can practice with items around your house. Close your eyes, and visualize something that you see every day in your house. Make sure it's something that you can visualize clearly and easily. Once you have that item clearly in your mind, play around with the color. If it's blue, change it from blue to green, and then red, then black, and so on. If you have difficulty with this, ask yourself:

"What would this xxx look like if it were navy blue with green polka dots?"

Our aim here is to create a full sensory experience. Remember, your subconscious mind does NOT know the difference between a "real" and imagined experienced. Anything that you visualize or imagine instantly becomes a memory.

What is the purpose of this exercise? Well, there are two purposes. One is to get you focused on the positive things that you want in your life, the things that will make it a little bit better, things that will actually make life more enjoyable. What's life if you can't have a little fun?

Two, this will help to activate the law of attraction in your favor. Basically, wherever you focus your attention is where you focus your energy and efforts.

In a nutshell, the thoughts we have in our minds vibrate at certain frequencies, depending on the thoughts we have. Regardless of the thought though, these thoughts will attract to us whatever it is that we focus on. For instance, if someone is constantly thinking about all the misery in the world, they will not only miss out on the beauty and wonder around them, but they will attract to themselves misery and suffering!!! I personally believe in this law, and I've seen it work in my favor many times. I've been sitting there hoping that so and so will call me and let me know if things have changed concerning xxx, and so and so and calls me.

Many people will tell you that all you have to do is sit back, visualize for about 20 minutes, and just wait for what you visualized to fall into your lap. Well, I don't think so. Let me tell you why: We have a physical body for a reason. If all you had to do was wish for something and have it materialize into existence, you wouldn't need a physical body.

You want to know what I think about visualizing? I think that visualizing simply focuses your attention on the desired outcome. The more frequently you visualize that outcome, the more you send the message to your subconscious mind that this is what you want. You are literally pushing yourself toward you goal by visualizing the desire outcome. Once you have the outcome clear in mind, then you do what is necessary to make it a reality.

In One school of thought, The Huna Religion, There are seven precepts or principles around which the system revolves, and are as follows:

The Seven Huna Principles

1: The World is What You Think It Is

Positive thoughts attract positive people and events, and negative thoughts attract negative people and events. I'm pretty sure you've seen this in your own life and situations. Some days, you tend to be surrounded by people who seem to have nothing about complaints about everything, and then some days you seem to be surrounded by people who are just in a good mood and happy to just be alive.

Corollary: Everything is a dream

Dreams are real and reality is a dream. The only test we use for a reality check is whether or not someone else experiences it. Hallucination means "your dream doesn't match my dream." "Reality" is a mass hallucination, or a shared dream. If this life is a dream and if we can wake up fully within it, then we can change the dream by changing our dreaming. Imagine what it would be like if you could dream yourself a whole new dream, different from the one that you currently take part in? What if you could dream up a brand new car or brand new place to live?

Corollary: All systems are arbitrary

All meanings are made up and the Absolute Truth is whatever you decide it is. What matters is how well the system works for you, not how true it is (which is an arbitrary concept).

2: There are No Limits

We experience two kinds of limitations: creative and filtered. Creative limitation assumes the purposeful establishment of limits within an infinite universe in order to create particular experiences, made by God or our own Higher Selves. These enable us to experience life as humans on Earth (to play by that particular set of rules - breaking the rules changes to another game). Filtered limitations are imposed by ideas and beliefs that inhibit creativity rather than enhance it, like beliefs that engender hopelessness, helplessness, revenge and cruelty. They generate focus without the potential for positive action.

Corollary: Everything is connected

The usual metaphor is a web of interdependence.

Corollary: Anything is possible

All you have to do is believe. However, because you are not alone in the Universe, the degree to which something can be shared depends on the beliefs of others around you.

Corollary: Separation is a useful illusion

Pure empathy makes you as helpless as the one suffering. Fear makes you lose sight of your role as dream weaver.

3: Energy Flows Where Attention Goes

Meditation and hypnosis are simply different techniques for doing the same thing - refocusing your attention toward more positive beliefs and expectations. As states, both are identical conditions of sustained focused attention. Those aspects of your present experience which seem enduring are the effect of habitual sustained focused attention carried on by your subconscious.

Corollary: Attention goes where energy flows

Attention is attracted to all kinds of high energy intensity.

Corollary: Everything is energy Thought is energy and one kind of energy can be converted into another kind of energy. NOW is the Moment of Power.

Karma exists and operates only in the present moment. It is your beliefs, decisions, and actions today about yourself and the world around you that give you what you have and make you what you are.

Thanks to memory we may carry over habits of body and mind from day to day, but each day is a new creation and any habit can be changed at any present moment - even if it isn't easy.

You select out of the immense resources of your gene pool those characteristics that best reflect your present beliefs and intentions. Your parents/social background have nothing to do with your present, but what you believe about them now and how you react to those beliefs does.

Corollary: Everything is relative

You define "now" based on your focus (second, hour, year, and lifetime).

Corollary: Power increases with sensory attention

Many people living today aren't even here - most of their attention is focused on the past or the future. To the degree they diminish their awareness of the present moment, their power and effectiveness in the present also decreases.

#4: To Love is to Be Happy With

Love exists to the degree that you are happy with the object of your love. The unhappy part comes from fear, anger and doubt. To be deeply in love means to be deeply connected, and the depth and clarity of the connection increases as fear, anger and doubt are removed.

Corollary: Love increases as judgment decreases

Criticism kills relationships; praise builds and rebuilds them. When you give praise you reinforce the good and it grows. When you criticize you reinforce the bad and it grows.

Corollary: Everything is alive, aware and responsive

Your subconscious takes any praise or criticisms it hears to heart, even if it's directed elsewhere, even if you're saying it. Each criticism separates you from and decreases your awareness of what you criticize, until you end up responding to a secondary creation of your own that may no longer resemble the original. When someone criticizes you, praise yourself to counteract it. All Power Comes From Within.

For every event that you experience you creatively attract it through your beliefs, desires, fears and expectations, and then react to it habitually or respond to it consciously. This does not mean that you are to blame for your abuse or injury, because you were probably not conscious of your negative beliefs, attitudes and expectations. It also does not mean the other person is innocent.

Corollary: Everything has power

You do not have ALL the power in the world - everyone has the same power. The good news - you can work with these powers. Corollary: Power comes from authority; Confident authority is the key to conscious creation.

Effectiveness is the Measure of Truth. The means determine the end, not the ends justify the means. What is really important is what works.

Corollary: There is always another way to do anything; every problem has more than one solution.

If the goal is important, you should never give up, just change your approach.

Take a moment and REALIZE the implications that it has. Could you imagine how much healthier you would be if you could focus on the positive things in life and focus on the good that may come of it? How much better and SMOOTHER would life run if we could JUST TAKE ONE of these principles, INTERNALIZE IT, and use it to help solve problems in our lives? Think about it.

Remember, we can only focus on one thing at a time, so how could you possibly be focused on something negative when you're focused on the positive or desired outcome? How easy would it be to WRITE DOWN A LIST of the things that we want in our life and look at that list every chance we get?

Simple breathing exercises for more energy and vitality

1. THE CLEANSING BREATH

Upon rising in the morning, stand by your window, and if you can, feel the warmth of the rising sun on your body as you breathe deeply. Hold the breath for about 2 seconds, and then release it. Continue this breathing pattern for as long as you wish, but don't be surprised if you make it half way to work and realize that you haven't had your morning cup of coffee.

Simply take a deep breath and allow your stomach to expand. Then, on the exhalation or release of the breath, suck in your stomach as though you wanted to touch your navel to your spine. This will ensure that you exhale the maximum amount of carbon dioxide, which is merely a waste product and serves no purpose in the body.

Other benefits of this true form of deep breathing include better digestion, more physical energy and stamina, and clearer thinking. AND IT'S ABSOLUTELY FREE!!! Can you ask for anything better than that? Nature has provided you with a virtually unlimited source of HEALTH and Vitality.

When you have adopted a habit of deep breathing, true and natural deep breathing, you can move on to more sophisticated breathing exercises, such as the "bellows breath". It's a form of breathing that is utilized in many forms of yoga, the purpose of which is to refresh the mind and body with life giving energy. Although it can be done while standing, it is advisable that you attempt this breathing while seated, as the rush of oxygen maybe too much for a beginner you may find yourself on the floor. Another variation on the cleansing breath is to increase the hold time gradually.

2. THE BELLOWS BREATH –

Sit comfortably with your spine upright and close your eyes. Exhale all the air from your lungs. Then begin deep in and out breathing through your nose silently. For the first twenty breaths take two second slow forceful inhalations and two second slow, forceful exhalations. It's easier to keep track of the number of breaths by counting on your fingers.

The next twenty breaths are performed faster with approximately one second inhalations and one second exhalations. These are also performed in through the nose, silently. Finally, perform twenty rapid bellows breaths, with approximately half second inhalations and half second exhalations. After the twenty rapid breaths, perform one more slow deep breath and then simply feel the sensations in your body. You will notice that your mind is clear and quiet while your body is energized.

Do not hyperventilate to the point where you are feeling lightheaded or dizzy. The breath movement is almost entirely abdominal, using your diaphragm to move air. Your head and shoulders should be relaxed and mostly still. Use bellows breathing when you are feeling a little sluggish and need a quick replenishment of energy. It's also something very good to do before you mediate, as it will help clear the drowsiness from your head and leave your mind bright and awake.

This happens to be my favorite form of breathing meditation as it provides me with quick energy and keeps me sharp and alert throughout the entire day, and my energy levels stays the same, depending on the stressors I'm stressing out about☺ The bellows breath is a good method to use when you want to energize yourself. Just remember to perform some other exercise if your goal is to have a sound night of sleep, otherwise you'll be awake for a good part of night. This in itself is not a bad thing, as you can use the energy generated by the breathing exercise to make plans for the next day or even next month. We live in a world where we have choice, so you can do as you wish.

HEALING YOURSELF AND OTHERS WITH A SMILE:)

It's natural to smile when we feel good about something or someone that we really enjoy being around. Have you ever been around somebody that made you feel so good that you just had to break out in the biggest cheesiest smile that you were capable of, even though you never understand what compelled you to smile? All you know is that you feel good whenever you're around this person and even though you don't smile outwardly, you feel as though your entire body, deep inside of you, is smiling. You feel warm.

Science may have some answers to the warm fuzzy feeling we've been getting.

There have multiple studies on the benefits of smiling and surprisingly, scientists and researchers discovered that smiling releases endorphins, the chemical that is responsible for making us feel good.

A smile not only has the power to make us feel good, but it also has the power to warm the hearts of others. Have you ever been feeling down when all of a sudden, stranger smiles at you, and for some reason unknown to you, you had to smile back? Smiling is contagious, almost hypnotic. When we smile at people, they can't help but to smile back. That's the way we human beings are wired. We unconsciously mirror each other. I'm known for being a friendly guy in my circle of friends, and I'm always extending my hand to people on the street, complete strangers. I know that whenever I extend my hand, the stranger to whom I've extended it often extends his in reciprocation, often to their utter surprise. It's something so simple, but people fail to realize the power of smiling. When you smile at others, they will smile back. It's as simple as that.

If you don't believe, the next time you're out and about, make a note to yourself that you will smile at 3 complete strangers today, with the intention that they feel good. This is very important. Have the intention in mind to make them feel good. If they don't smile back, that's fine. A smile is totally free and you can keep giving them as long as you are breathing. A smile has the power to change lives, when applied at the proper moment. When you look into someone's eyes and smile, you acknowledge that they exist and you energize them.

A smile can make the lonely feel better and brighten up their day. The power of smiling is something that you should use every day and can use right now. The next time you see someone that might be down or feeling blue, just make eye contact with them and smile. Watch the magic happen.

The "inner smile" technique is a means of using the power of smiling to help your body stay healthy and vibrant.
It's very simple and you can do it anytime you feel as if you need a pick me up or boost, without having to resort to all that coffee. This is obviously something that you want to do when you're by yourself and not driving, as that could be dangerous :)

All you do is close your eyes, and relax your body as completely as you are able to at the moment.

Scientists discovered that when we close our eyes, something very special happens: Our brainwaves slow down and we enter what is commonly known as ALPHA brainwave. It's characterized by brainwaves that cycle ten times per second. It's the level of activity in which we daydream and the point at which our imaginations come to life. 20 minutes at alpha brainwave is the equivalent of 6 hours of deep sleep!!

Now, take a deep breath and hold it for a few seconds, and the let it out through your mouth. Do this breathing pattern five times. Breathing in this manner activates the natural built in relaxation response we have. Being relaxed is crucial to being vibrant and healthy. Tension leads to all manner of diseases, believe it or not.

Once you feel relaxed, simply smile. Smile as broadly and widely as you are able, since no one is around, you can smile as widely as you like.

Smile this way for a moment, and when you feel ready, I want you to focus your attention on your chest area, the area where you heart is. As you smile, continue to sense that heart area and notice what you feel.

When you feel ready to move one, smile as you focus on the area of your solar plexus. Notice what you feel in this area.
That's it. That's all there is to it. You might notice that you feel a bit different.

You can perform this meditation in your bed before you go to sleep. Smile as you focus your attention to the major organs in your body. Smile down to your legs; smile to your back, your neck, your butt, every part of your body deserves the warmth of a smile. As you smile to each spot on your body, tell it "Thank You!" mind body communication just doesn't flow from your body to your mind; you can flow it from your mind to your body. Your body will glow with warmth and vitality.

Studies have been done that demonstrate that when you focus your attention on a certain part of your body, you stimulate the nerves in that area that's being focused upon. Your thoughts have the ability to light up your nerves. Smiling to your body turns it on, so to speak.

BEING AWAKE: MORE THAN HAVING YOUR EYES OPEN

It occurred to me as I'm writing this book that people today are awake for the most part, but not alert. By alert, I mean that we don't realize what is going on around us. We fail to pay attention to the activities taking place around us. How many times have you been walking around the mall, looking for a particular store, only to realize that you can't find the store because you you've already walked past it, not once, but twice!!!

Well, what happen was that most likely, as you were walking around the mall, your attention was drawn to something going on in your immediate area or to some problem or situation going on in your life right now. Well, remember that since the mind is indivisible, we can only focus on one thing at a time. While you were thinking about whatever you were thinking about, your attention was so totally absorbed by it that you failed to see the store that you were looking for.

I used to have that same problem: I was so absorbed in what was going on in my own head that I didn't even notice what was going on around me. It was a real problem, as my daily life started to suffer since I could not focus my attention outward and perform effectively.

After much research, I found an answer to my dilemma, and it was staring me in the face the entire time: In order to focus my attention outward, outside of my head, I needed to be focused on what was going on around me. DUH!!!

Whenever I find myself "trapped in my head", I simply focus my attention on something that out in front of me, with my physical eyes. I pick a spot in front of me and just focus my attention on it completely. It's a simple trick, but it works wonders for me, and it will work for you as well.

The next time you find yourself distracted by some problem or situation in your life, just pick a spot in front of you somewhere and focus your complete attention on it. You do this as long as you like, since we naturally have to focus outward in our daily life. It's simple, yet powerfully effective.

Another simple yet very effective way to get in touch with the world around you is to simply pay attention to the information that your senses is providing you.

What do you hear?

What do you smell?

What do you feel?

Actually touch the things around you (don't touch people unless you have their permission though :). When you touch things, notice how they feel. It's a very simple way to wake you and cause you to be alert, ready to do the things you need to accomplish for that day.

Allow yourself to really focus on the sounds and sights around you. When you reach out and touch something in your environment, how does it feel against your fingers? Is it rough? Is it soft? Being highly aware of your sense of touch has benefits that pay off in other...situations. Use your imagination. Imagine how much more fun you'll have with your partner as you run your newly sensitized fingers through their hair or brush their cheek with the back of your hand. Just imagine how much more fun you'll have... Think of the possibilities...

A SIMPLE ACUPRESSURE TECHNIQUE TO REDUCE STRESS AND FEAR!!!

Have you ever been out somewhere and all of a sudden for one reason or another, you start to get really nervous, and then that nervousness grows into fear, uncontrollable fear that literally paralyzes you and stops you doing what you need to do to accomplish your goals and desires? Well, get in line because I know that feeling all too well. It's as if someone is literally holding you in place, only, that person who's holding you back is YOU. It's not intentional; over the course of our lives, we develop defense mechanisms that have positive intentions that protect us from being hurt. Well actually, it's a response called the fight of flight response. There's also a lesser known response called the freeze response, which seems to be a common reaction to fear. This reaction is built into us over centuries to help protect us from less-than-friendly environments.

What seems to happen is that we have certain thoughts about situations and those thoughts almost always tend to be about what could go wrong in the situation. The more negative outcomes you imagine or expect, the more the feeling of fear seems to increase. You're literally stacking this fear up with each negative outcome you've visualized.

What would it be like if you could imagine clearly a positive outcome to that upcoming situation or event? What if you were to imagine giving that presentation successfully, fully relaxed and fully confident, confident because you know your stuff, and you can explain it to everybody in the room in a way that they completely understand. See the interested look on your listener's faces as they are eager to hear every word that you say. What would that be like?

Well, there's something you can do about it. With this simple technique, you can even reprogram yourself to act normally in situations where you would normally break into a sweat and breathe heavily. It's so simple that when I came across it 4 years ago, I didn't believe, because it seemed to be TOO damn simple. But it works and this one little technique has improved the quality of my life IMMENSELY. I can things today where a year ago I would literally have a panic attack. It worked for me and it can work for you.

Here it is: There's a small pressure point on the back of your hand, on the top of your hand between the tendons of your little finger and your ring finger. It's the fleshy part right there in between those two tendons. This point is used in oriental medicine to relieve feelings of fear and anxiety. Once you've reprogrammed your mind and body to relax in trying situations, then you can visualization and affirmation to program yourself to react in the way that YOU choose to react.

Here's the technique: The next time you feel fearful, find someplace quiet to go to and tap that spot on the back of your hand as breath in deeply through your nose and let the breath out through your mouth. Continue tapping and breathing in this way until your feel different. Believe me, you'll know it when it happens. In fact, you might even want to put your book down right now and practice this simple technique.

Whenever you feel fearful about some upcoming event or situation, use this technique and notice the difference. Over time, your body will react less and less to that stressful situation until your reach the point where you no longer have any emotional reaction to that stressful thought or feeling. Once you reach that point where you feel indifferent, you can then use techniques like affirmations and auto suggestion and self hypnosis to program yourself to act the way you want to act in any situation. Let me add that this isn't a cure for fear, but it does help to take the edge off.

A SIMPLE PROCESS FOR FALLING ASLEEP EFFORTLESSLY!!!

Now, I know how hard it can be to fall asleep at night, especially after you've had a trying day at work, or you just had a stressful day in general handling the challenges in your life. I've had night where I could not sleep, despite the fact that I exercise regularly. It just seems like even though your body is extremely tired, your mind is chattering away, replaying the events of the day and worrying about the challenges that you'll have to deal with tomorrow.

Well, the reason this happens is because when we think, all of our attention and energy is focused in our heads, where we have our thoughts. Our heads are filled with different thoughts, all of which are vying for your attention to them. They call thoughts "fleeting" for a reason.

What if I told you there was a way to fall asleep and stop that chattering in your head? Well, here's a simple process for falling asleep effortlessy and sleeping deeply and soundly. Imagine what it would be like if you could fall asleep like this EVERY NIGHT and wake up feeling as though you've been totally rejuvenated, ready to tackle the challenges waiting for you that day.

Here's what I do when I have trouble falling asleep because I have too much energy in my head:

The first thing I make sure to do is to turn off the ringer on my phone. This ensures that I sleep deeply and peacefully with no interruptions, except perhaps for the occasional bathroom trip☺ If there's an emergency, I can be reached via my cell phone or police escort. I go downstairs and get warm up some milk. What I do is get some milk, usually full fat milk, and I warm it up in a pot for about five minutes. I don't want the milk to be scalding; I just want it warm enough to drink comfortably. As the milk heats up on the stove, there's usually a film that develops on the surface. Just use a spoon or fork and pick up that film and toss it away. Heating the milk denatures, or breaks down, the protein molecules so my body can absorb them easier.

One thing that people don't know is that in India, warm milk and honey is frequently prescribed as a cure to impotence. The warm milk and honey increase the amount of semen in your testicles generate. Believe me when I tell you this; I just don't take people's word for things. Long story short, I gave it a shot for about a week and it works.

Once the milk is warm enough to drink, but not hot enough to burn me, I add some honey to it. I grab a banana and eat that with my milk. The banana has tryptophan in it, the same chemical in turkey that causes you to fall asleep. Have you ever had an incredible Thanksgiving Day dinner, and despite the festive atmosphere, you just feel sleepy for some reason? That's the tryptophan in the turkey which causes that.

I head upstairs and make sure all the light are off and no light can enter my bedroom. Any type of light will cause your body to decrease its production of melatonin, a chemical that's released in total darkness and necessary for health and vitality. After I've enjoyed my milk and banana, I lay down in bed.

Once I'm in a comfortable position, I mentally say to myself: "Whatever has to be done tomorrow has to wait until tomorrow. I want to sleep deeply and peacefully now.... I'll deal with everything tomorrow." I usually repeat this a couple of times, as a way of telling my subconscious mind my intentions. Repetition is very powerful and our subconscious minds respond to it powerfully.

I lay down in bed and I place my hands on the spot under my belly button. I make sure to place my right hand over my left hand. I'm placing my hand over my second chakra, or energy center. What this does is to help draw all that energy – and your attention - down from your head and back into your body, while at the same time it totally relaxes your body.

As I lay there like that, I take three deep breaths, in through the nose and out through the mouth. This type of breathing automatically reduces the stress you have inside you. It helps you to trigger the relaxation response.

You want to sleep peacefully and deeply, and everything else can wait until tomorrow.

Now, I focus my attention on my body and I become aware of all the sensations that I'm feeling. I just sit there and watch the sensations and notice all the sensations that make themselves known.

Before I know it, it's the next morning, and I always wake up feeling like I've been asleep for three days, always feeling fresh and I literally wake up out of bed and stretch.

Please don't underestimate the importance of sleeping deeply, because it's during sleep that our bodies repair us. Always arrange your schedule so that you get everything done by at least 6 or 7 in the afternoon, that way you can go home and relax and get ready for sleep.

Some other things that really help with sleeping, I've found, are:

1) No exercise at least 2 hours before I have to go to sleep. Exercise is stimulating and releases

adrenaline, which is something you don't need if you're trying to go to sleep. There are times, however, when you just need to tire yourself out completely before you can sleep peacefully. Everybody is different, so you may need to exercise vigorously whereas another person can just relax and release all tension. See what works for you.

2) If I've really had a challenging day, I do the fear tap that I mentioned earlier in this book, and as I tap, I breathe deeply in through my nose and out through my mouth, as I mentally tell myself " Everything's safe, I'm okay"

3) Stretching is excellent for releasing stress that has accumulated during the course of the day. Any basic yoga exercise will do. The one that I perform regularly is the "sun salutation", which is very excellent for relaxation. As a matter of fact, you can stretch all throughout your day. If you work at a desk, you can stretch as you get up or sit in your chair. You see people doing it all the time. It's the body's way of relaxing us.

4) I have my last meal two hours before I go to sleep. Digestion

   is a process that takes a lot of energy, and it can keep you

   from getting that deep, recuperative sleep that you need to be

   the best you can be for the next day. Remember, it's during

   sleep that our bodies regenerate. Any energy that it has to

   divert towards digestion is energy that is not being used to

   heal you. During sleep, our body does amazing things, one of

   which is the removal of dead cells and potentially cancerous

   tumors. This is why a small snack like warm milk and a

   banana are optimal for getting revitalizing sleep.

I write out list of all the things that needs to be done tomorrow

and I write them out in the order in which they need to be done.

This is a way of reassuring me that these things will be done and

there is no need to mull over them in my sleep. I write down

everything I can think off and I put that list in my coat pocket so

that I make sure I have when I need it the following day. As a

matter of fact, I set everything up ahead of time: I get my shoes

out and my clothes and lay them out on a chair or my dresser

drawer. Then I go downstairs and make sure that I have my

readymade lunch prepared which consists of tons of fruits and nuts and some protein. By preparing my own lunch, I have control of two things:

That I have the optimal nutrients to keep my mind and body functioning all day.

That I can make more efficient use of my time, time that would have been spent going back and forth to some local restaurant, can now be used to sit and eat in silence while ideas just seem to come to me. I highly recommend that you consider this practice of setting things up ahead of time so that you can literally roll out of bed and begin the day.

I usually meditate before I go to sleep, to help clear your mind even further and deeper. It's nothing fancy or mystical; I just sit upright in a comfortable chair (not a recliner, I'd fall asleep and the purpose is to stay awake and notice what's floating through my head). I relax and take some deep breaths. Yeah, I know that I mention breathing a lot, but the benefits of breathing are nearly infinite. Did you know that cancer cannot survive in an oxygen rich environment or in other words, a body that is routinely saturated with oxygen through exercise? I also make sure that the window is cracked a bit if the weather permits, as the brain needs lots of oxygen to function at its optimal capacity and crank out those ideas that can generate serious amounts of income.

I just sit there and notice what I'm feeling in my body and I also pay attention to the thoughts floating through my head. I also make every effort to relax my body progressively, by focusing on each body part and telling it to relax, and as I tell it to relax, I take a really deep breath and let it out through the mouth. The goal is TOTAL relaxation.

A hot bath is always helpful. Running bath water and sitting down in it for about 20 minutes is an excellent way to relax and an incredible way to kick start your way to an awesome night of sleep. I make sure that I take a hot bath every night, so that I can relax and shut my eyes. In the privacy of my own bathroom, I find that it's a quite relaxing experience and I always feel better after I step out of that water. It feels as if the water has absorbed all the negative energy that I've accumulated throughout the course of my day. I even tell myself that all that negative energy is going down the drain with the water. I make sure that I tell myself that what's going outside of these bathroom doors is not my concern for the time being, unless it is a genuine emergency.

One very inexpensive and tasty way I've discovered through research to fall asleep quickly is to eat some cherries. Yes, you've heard me right. Cherries help your body produce more melatonin, a hormone released during sleep that is partly responsible for the rejuvenating effects of deep, restful sleep. So the next time you find yourself having a hard time going to sleep, just run down to your local supermarket and grab a bagful of cherries. Who knows, you may run into the love of your life or find the answer to a situation that's been plaguing you. Cherries are one of the few known food sources of melatonin, a potent antioxidant produced naturally by the body's pineal gland that helps regulate biorhythm and natural sleep patterns.

Scientists have found melatonin-rich tart cherries (commonly enjoyed as dried, frozen, juice or concentrate) contain more of this powerful antioxidant than what is normally produced by the body. Eating cherries can be a natural way to boost your body's melatonin levels to hasten sleep and slow down the aging process.

Progressive relaxation is a process that's deceptively simple yet incredibly effective. It's so simple that sometimes just doing progressive relaxation will allow you to drift off into dreamland. Simply tense and relax your muscles alternately. Flex your calves by pointing your toes upwards. Hold this tension for about five seconds, and then relax. Do the same with every other part of your body and relax. Make sure you pay careful attention to your arms and legs, as they are your extremities and your body naturally sends blood to them as we use them quite frequently.

Speaking of anger, there's a simple way to control your anger. It's so simple that you probably wouldn't believe unless you actually tried it. The secret is to…. Stay completely still!!! Yes, I said stay completely still. Anger and tension go hand in hand, so it makes sense that if you tense, then you're more prone to get angry, but if you completely relax your arms and allow that relaxation to spread to all you limbs, then I guarantee you that you will have a hard time getting angry. I had a hard time believing it myself, until I gave it a shot. I simply relax my arms and then take a deep breath. I find that my anger diminishes greatly and I can confront the situation in a relaxed state of mind. You have to realize that we are in complete control of our bodies so it has to obey us. It's a simple as that. The pain we sometime feel is good, because it lets us know there's a problem.

You can try it right now: Think of something that really ticks you off. Got it? Good, now, relax your arms and legs completely as you think of that incident. Notice your feelings.

Please notice that I spent A LOT of time and effort on this one chapter. Do you know why I spent so much time on this chapter? I spent a lot of time on this chapter because I truly believe that sleeping deeply and soundly is something that money cannot buy, no matter how much of it you may have accumulated. Nothing can buy that feeling of absolute comfort and peace of knowing that you can control how your life turns out; Nothing can buy that feeling of lying in bed and knowing that you can sleep deeply because you now have the energy and willingness to handle all situations that come your way, no matter how big they may appear to be.

I personally believe that there are no big or small situations, only the reactions to them are big or small. A situation is nothing more than a situation, and event to which we attach excess emotional energy. Have you ever heard of the term "blowing things out of proportion"? Well there's some validity in the saying. Because all too often, we tend to make things much more difficult than they really need to be. By blowing things out of proportion, we give what should be a challenge so much energy that it grows into something we lack the capacity to handle. Remember how earlier I mentioned that energy follows your attention? Well, emotion generates energy, so imagine how much you would be feeding a situation when you are panicked, upset, or scared?

I'm not saying that you should deny your situations out of existence; I'm saying that you need to acknowledge the situation in all of its detail. Once you know the situation for what it is, then you can work on coming up with solutions to changing it.

A SIMPLE WAY TO FAST WITHOUT EVEN TRYING!!!

I don't know how many of you know anything about fasting, but it's essentially taking a break from eating while your body diverts its energy to rejuvenating your wonderful body. Your enzyme pool has a chance to replenish itself. Normally, we eat so much during the day that our body's energies are solely dedicated to digesting our food, whereas it could be directing that energy to the removal of toxins and waste material for the body.

What if I told you that we naturally fast for seven hours or more per day? Would you believe it? Well, if you don't, believe it!!! Every night when you sleep, your body is going eight hours or more without food. During this time, your body has to find sustenance, so it has no choice but to turn to the waste material inside your body. In the process of devouring this unwanted waste material, it cleans up your blood stream. This includes eating any masses of material that shouldn't be in there, including cells that could become cancerous/already are.

Another really amazing process that occurs in your body while you sleep is the release of Growth Hormone, or GH. Your body releases its highest amounts of this substance when you're in your deepest sleep cycle, the delta brainwave cycle. Delta brainwave is complete unconsciousness. GH is responsible for the building of new tissue in your body, like muscles and organs. By becoming aware of this nightly phenomenon, you can take simple steps to maximize your output and experience faster lean mass gains:

1) Throw High Intensity Play Sequences (HIPS) into EVERY one of training session, whether your focus for the day is resistance training or cardiovascular training. Discover your heart rate ranges (see the appendices for complete details) to help yourself design suitable HIPS for your body and current fitness levels. Not only will you be strengthening your heart; you'll also achieve levels of intensity that will allow you to release more GH.

2) Go to bed on an empty stomach. Being fasted with an empty stomach will allow your body to take full advantage of the GH surge that you get during deep sleep. If you can't go to sleep on an empty stomach, then make sure that you last meal is low is sugar, high in protein, and high in fat. Eating

foods that meet these criteria will keep you full until you hit your deep states of sleep, at which point its smooooth sailing into fat burning.

3) Don't waste your time in the gym doing single joint exercises; instead, focus your attention on multi-joint exercises. Not only will you burn more calories, but you also elicit a greater response of GH. Your single joint movements should be performed AFTER you've done all of your multi joint movements. This order of training helps improve athletic performance by helping you avoiding unnecessary muscle fatigue, which can hinder your muscle efficiency. You don't just want a body that looks great; you also want your body to perform awesome.

4) Avoid white bread/pasta; instead, eat only vegetables, fruits, and grains (if your stomach allows for grains). Multigrain usually means high fiber, which means longer digestion, which means you slooooooww done the release of insulin dramatically. All of this means that you keep your body in a state of optimal energy AND GH output. If you're worried that eating at night will set you back (you shouldn't be),

then get up, walk around the house, find a spot to relax and do the following:

a) Take 5 deep breaths, inhaling for 5 seconds, holding for 5 seconds, and then releasing for a count of 5.

b) March in place for 1-2 minutes as you breathe deeply.

c) Notice if you're still hungry. If you're not, then hit the sack and sweet dreams!!

5) Make sure that you're eating the right amounts of self-body friendly protein for YOUR body and your life activities. Lean muscle needs source material AND GH to grow, so give your body both. As everyone has different bio-individuality, the amounts of protein I eat won't benefit you and the same goes for me. In general, a good serving size of protein for most people is about the size of YOUR palm, NOT Shaq's, got it?

Like I mentioned earlier, your body is amazing and protects you even while you sleep. In a natural healthy state of mind and body, you should literally be rolling out of bed, ready to meet the day, filled with energy and expectation, expectation that this day is going to be something incredible. I feel that way almost every morning, and I want the people who read this book to apply this information and feel that way every day, so that you can go out and make other people feel good.

HELPING THE PEOPLE THAT YOU CARE ABOUT

One thing that really helps me to get out of bed in the morning and live life is the fact that I'm in a position to help my friends and family. I can help them and I want to help them because I love them and I want to see them accomplish their goals and lives their lives to fullest extent of which they are capable. I really feel that this should a sub-goal that everyone sets for themselves: to help friends and family as much as you are able to. As much as is within your power, at least.

Frequently, my friends and family come to me with problems in school or in the personal lives or just because they need somebody to listen to them. I make sure that I listen carefully to what they are telling me, and then I help them as best I can. I make sure that I ask for clarification on anything that's not completely clear to me. By doing this, I covertly get them to focus in on the real issue that they are having. I give them advice that they can easily take action on and change the situation to a better one.

I think that simply being someone that people can come to for advice is a simple, but powerful way to help the ones that you love and care about and want to see do good in this world. Even complete strangers come up to me asking me for advice, and believe it or not, I appreciate the fact that they approach me, because it gives me a chance to at least make one persons' day better than it was before we met. The thing that I hear the most from strangers is that they always feel better after talking through their problems.

When a stranger approaches who doesn't have a machine gun or is brandishing a shiny bowie knife, and if you have the time to do so, talk with them. You may actually learn something from the interaction. I've learned so much from complete strangers that it's ridiculous.

I personally believe that one of the keys to vibrant health and vitality is having relationships that flow smoothly, in which everyone listens to each other and understands each other. There are many ways to do this, but do this you MUST if you want your relationships to prosper. Imagine how much more amazing your life would be if all of your relationships strived and everyone involved was happy and fulfilled?

One very simple way to do this is to PAY ATTENTION!!! I know you might be screaming, "DUH!!!", but, many people don't realize that there's an effective way to pay attention, one which allows everyone involved to feel like they've been actually heard.

When you are speaking with someone, focus on the words they use to describe things. The words that people use determine how they experience the world. In Neurolinguistic programming, these are called "representational systems".

We experience the world in sensory terms. I'm pretty sure you know somebody who is always talking about their feelings, or the person who just doesn't "see" something happening, or the person who "hears you loud and clear"? Well, these are representational systems and you can use them to gain a deeper rapport with people, sometimes on levels that you might have initially thought to be impossible.

The next time you're talking with someone, pay close attention to the sensory terms they utilize frequently. This will give an idea of their representational system. For an even more precise way to uncover their representational system, ask them this question:

"What something exciting that you did recently?"

Listen to the sensory language they use and you'll uncover their representational system.

Don't stop there though: Once you've identified their sensory language, begin to slowly speak to them in their language. Speak in the sensory terms that they use. Notice how they respond to you.

You'll have deeper rapport just by using this one strategy.

How could you use this information in your daily life?

At work?

At home?

In meeting people?

For what I consider to be an incredible book on how to influence people positively, you might want to buy Dale Carnegie's book "How to win friends and influence people". This book is my bible and I frequently refer to it when I want to meet people or when I'm entering new social situations.

The End… Or is It?!?!?!?

I like to conclude by saying that I really appreciate your taking the time to read this book and I know that if you even apply just one of these simple tactics daily, the quality of your life will improve dramatically. The key word here is: "Apply".

I've provided you with space on the back of each page so that you can write down any thoughts or ideas that come to your mind. You know yourself better than anyone else on the planet.

If you need inspiration, rip the pages out of the book and pin them up on your wall, so that they are in plain sight and you always have a reminder, something to keep you focused on your goals. You see children do it all the time: They put up posters of people that the really admire. The ancient Greeks were firm believers in this. Pregnant Greek women would surround themselves with statues and images of the gods and goddesses they felt closest to, as they believed that the images would impact upon them daily and the child that was to come into the world would take the image of the gods. Really makes you think about the versatility and adaptability of the human body, doesn't it? I also think that this practice would go a long way to explain why the children of couples often times are born favoring someone other than the two parents....:)) HAHAHAHAHA

Here's a simple tip for you college students that may be reading this: How to study effectively. This goes for all you book readers who study for personal issues. Make sure you have food that conducive to studying, food that energizes your mind. Make sure that you have lots and lots of fruit, as fruit contains natural sugars that the brain uses to work with. No candy, until you're finished. If possible, you can put a "do not disturb" sign on your door. You need total focus and concentration so that you can comprehend what the author is saying: First and foremost, you need to state your intention either aloud or mentally to yourself. This is a way to focus your attention, to make it laser sharp.

Before I read a book, I always tell myself that "I'm going to read this book and take notes on it. I'm going to focus my complete attention on this book so that I can understand the author clearly, so that I can use this information to better myself, etc" Your statement of intent doesn't have to be so involved, just so long as you have an intention to sit down and read and take notes.

1) Turn off the TV, Phone and Radio. Plug everything out except for the lights. These things in the background will only distract you. I know firsthand that when I'm working to get something done, having the television playing in the background constantly draws my attention to what's in the television, when my attention should be here in the NOW, focusing on getting that book done.

2) Get out your pen and paper and get comfortable, whatever that means to you. Make sure you are sitting up, as lying down is typically associated with sleep. Your subconscious mind is programmed to go to sleep when you lie down. This is one of the main reasons that meditation experts want their students to either sit cross legged or sit up: because your need to be awake to get the benefits. So sit up in a comfortable chair and read away. Cross legged sitting isn't too comfortable for most people, so sitting upright with legs uncrossed is preferred by most.

3) As you read something, take the time to really understand the point the author wants to get across. If possible, write out his/her point in YOUR OWN WORDS. This helps to make the understanding your own, since you have to focus to really understand what's being said. Think of what you're reading from this viewpoint: you're actually reading the author's thoughts and beliefs, written on paper/kindle.

4) Dedicate at least one hour to one particular subject a night/day. This is really simple to do and you can easily

find a way in your daily routine to make it happen.

Remember, your education is important; it's going to be the

thing that gets you all those high paying jobs so you can live

out all those dreams you have floating around in your head. If

you want to, that is☺

5) When you feel as though your head can't take in any more

information, simply stop what you're doing, open a window

if desirable, take 5 or six deep breaths, and then do the ear

tug I mentioned earlier. In addition to waking up you up in

the morning, it also clears out your head and opens your

mind, so that you can take in more information.

6) When you're done studying, stand up and stretch out,

breathing deeply as you do.

Use this formula for studying whenever you like.

Breaking people out of negative states

It's so simple to break people out of their negative states that you wouldn't believe it. The next time you encounter somebody in a bad mood, all you have to do is walk up them and ask them a weird question or ask them for the time. This works because asking questions causes people to stop thinking about what they were thinking about before and focus their attention outside themselves. When they are finished externalizing their awareness, then they have to go back into themselves and figure out what they were thinking about before. Often times, they completely forget what they were thinking about, depending on how deeply they were associated into that state.

The End… Again.

I really enjoyed writing this for you and I know that you enjoyed reading it since you've made it this far☺ If there's any questions or comments that you have floating in your mind, then please feel free to email me at and I will do my best to answer your questions or direct you to the resources necessary to answer your questions:

I want to leave you with these words, words that help me daily to focus my attention and energy on the right things for me:

Material things are good, because we live in a material world, but the growth and development of your mind and spirit matter more than anything else, because these things are eternal, as is the human spirit. When we go from this material plane, we only carry with us the feelings we have and the lessons that we learned. Live a life that you truly want to live. There's more than enough for everyone.

Regrets are pointless, because we can't go back in time. On the physical plane. We can learn from our mistakes, however. We can travel back and forth in our imagination. You do it every day. It's called "memory". When you "travel forward" or think about the possibilities, then it's called "imagination" or fantasy. Why not go back in time and remember pleasant times? Why not imagine what it would be like if you were living your perfect life? Just seems to make sense when you stop and really think about it, wouldn't you agree? When you realize how powerfully your imagination can help shape the life you want experience, then you automatically start to feel a sense of gratitude and awe.

Thank you and remember to breathe deeply, wherever you find yourself. Pull that air down in to your stomach area, know that you are breathing the life force, and it's totally free!!! When all else fails, find some place where you can be alone, and breath in deeply, hold for a few seconds, and then exhale. Do these until you feel a little better.

Nobody is perfect and we all have our moments, moments when we get angry or sad. The trick is learning how to deal with these incidents and emotions in a productive manner and consciously deciding to change our state from negative back to positive. Every time we lose control, we get a glimpse of what's going on inside of us and we also get feedback on the areas that we need to work on developing. Anger can be powerful fuel to get stuff done. It's usually when we're angry or just plain tired of a certain situation that we make potential powerful decisions.

When you give a gift, hold it close to you and imagine how much enjoyment the recipient will gain from it.

So, take what you learn from this book and make the changes in your life that you need to make. Start small and see how each change impacts your life. The worst thing that could happen is that you actually learn something...)

LIVE A VIBRANT AND RADIANT LIFE!!!!

PS. GET A MINITRAMPOLINE!!!!

Bibliography:

1) Bates, William H. (md), *Better eyesight without Glasses*, New York, Henry Holt and Company, 1940, 1981

2) Eden and Feinstein, *Energy Medicine*, Penguin Group, New York, 1998

3) Chopra, Deepak, *Ageless Body, Timeless Mind*, Harmony Books, New York, 1993

4) Mckenzie, Eleanor, *The Joseph H. Pilates Method At home*, Ulysses Press, California

5) Roizen/ Mehmet, *You: The Owners Manual*, Harper Collins, New York, 2005

6) Aerobics and Fitness Association of America, *Aerobics: Theory And Practice*, HDL Publishing Company, California, 1985, 1988

7) Aurelius, Marcus, *The Meditations*, Hackett Publishing Company, Indianapolis, 1983

8) Benson, Stuart, *The Wellness Book: The comprehensive Guide to Maintaining Health and Treating Stress Related illness*, Simon and Schuster, New York, 1992

9) Eden, Donna, *Energy Medicine for Women*, Penguin Group, New York, 2008

10) Frost, Robert, *Applied Kinesiology*,

11) Carter, Albert E., The *Miracles Of Rebound Exercise*, The national institute of Reboundology and Health, Inc., Washington

12) Macrae, Janet, *Therapeutic Touch: A practical guide*, Alfred A. Knopf, New York, 1996

13) King, Serge, ***Urban Shaman***, 1990

Appendices

How to find your Specific Optimal Heart Zones ™ for Optimal Fat Burning!

Finding your max heart rate and optimal cardio zones

Note: EVERY training day dedicated to cardiovascular training MUST include a warm-up at your lower SOHZ's. Jumping to the higher zones without warming up your heart muscle properly is like taking your car from 0 to 70 without warming it up in the winter time. You could blow the engine. Or your heart. You've been warned.

FYI: For the law enforcement reading this, I don't condone going from 0 to 70. It's a hypothetical...

Before you venture forth into this section, please be aware that I'm going to disclaim you now☹:

As every one of you reading this is a bio INDIVIDUAL, like all things in life, this requires you to do some tweaking and playing around to get the numbers right for YOU. Become totally interested in your body and how it works and you will see how fun Purposeful Activity can be.

Consider these figures as a guideline from which you can design your own perfect Optimal Lifefit Program ©

Oh, and I don't take any responsibility or liability for heart explosions.

Get cleared by your medical doctor before you attempt this or any other fitness programs.

If you're going to become your own personal trainer, then you have to know how to calculate your own Specific Optimal Heart Zones © so you can get the most benefit from your fitness program.

I'll talk briefly about the purpose of cardiovascular training and why you may have been doing it wrong. It's ok; you have to know where you are right now before you can know which way to go, right?

Right.

In my experience and my not-so-humble-opinion. The purpose of a structured cardiovascular training program serves 4 primary purposes:

1) To help maintain the strength of your heart and lungs
2) To strengthen your heart muscle itself
3) To maintain a desired body composition, desired meaning the body YOU want, not the one your friends and family think you should have.
4) To increase good cholesterol levels so that your body has good source material from which to create powerful hormones like testosterone and DHEA.

If you're like most people wanting to change your body, you just hop on a piece of fitness equipment and walk/ ellipt until you've burnt your target amount of calories. That's fine, however, there's much more efficient way to do that. We have the capacity to burn either carbs or fats; the optimal way to burn them is to tap both.

Too much cardio training will increase your body's production of

Stress hormones like Cortisol, which will cause your body to break

into muscle tissue to use that for energy.

To become more efficient in your training sessions and burn more

calories with less work, you have to find your OHZ's. In order to do

this, you're going to need a calculator and something to record your

results on:

1) Subtract your age from 220
   I.e. 220- 35 = 185

2) The resulting number is your MAX Heart Rate zone. That's the max that I can get my heart rate up, close to the verge of exploding yet still keeping a smile on my face. We're not done yet though.

3) Take the resulting number and multiply it by the following percentages below:

a) 60%
b) 70%
c) 80%
d) 90%

4) When you've done this for each number, you should have a sheet of paper that looks like this:

a) 111 b) 129 c) 148 d) 166.5

So you have your heart rate zones… now how do you use them?
Simple:

The 1st and 2nd SOHZ'S are your fat burning zones. In order to burn body fat, you want to maintain your heart rate in these zones of intensity for a set period of time. You may find that your warm up period keeps you in these zones, which is perfect. In these zones, you're primary source of energy is fat.

The 3rd SOHZ is higher intensity. For me, I'm working / playing in my anaerobic glycotic zone, meaning that I'm relying heavily on both my anaerobic and aerobic energy systems to produce energy to help me complete my task. In this zone, I'm primarily using carbohydrates and glycogen for energy

The 4th zone is my true high intensity zone. At this point, my muscles burn and my heart wants to burst out of my chest and slap mah momma!

Depending on the outcomes you have for your fitness program, you're going to spend more time training in one zone than the other. HOWEVER, if you want to be totally fit and healthy, then you want to achieve each of these SOHZ'S as often as you can. Here's how:

1) The 1st and 2nd SOHZ'S are your Gateway Zones, which prepare your nervous system and muscles to achieve the higher zones. Because these are lower intensity zones, you can safely spend lots of time swimming playfully in them. You'll be tapping into fat stores and liberating them for future use. As these zones are technically warm-up Zones, you want to spend at least 6 minutes playing around in them.

2) The 3rd zone is where the fun starts. Because of its higher intensity nature, you want to spend small amounts of time playing here. This can be anywhere from 10 – 30 seconds, depending on your fitness levels and your goals. Here's the cool thing though:

You can always swim back to the 1st and 2nd zones for recovery. Once you're breath has slowed down a bit, you can jump right back into the middle end and play again. Repeat as much as you like☺

3) This 4th zone is the one that awesomely sucks. This is your highest safest SOHZ that you can reach. The time spent playing here is even shorter, 10- 20 seconds depending on your current fitness level and goals.

From this zone and all the other zones, you always swim safely back to your fat burning zones for recovery and here's the reasons why:

1) In your life, you NEVER stop. You are always growing and changing, new cells are being created within and old cells are being pooped out by skin and butthole, and possibly pee-pee hole.

2) Coming to a complete stop is dangerous, because you muscles help the heart do its work. When you stop moving, the blood starts pooling in the lower extremities, which means the heart gets very little help. This is bad if you are starting off training with a weak heart muscle. When you come out of the higher zones, walk in your

lower zones, even lower if necessary, to recover your

breath rhythm. March in place. Do jumping jacks. Keep

moving until your heart rate gets back to your low SOHZ.

Appendix 2:

10 supplements to help you Burn Fat Faster!

Before you read on, please make sure that you check with your

doctor before you take any of the supplements listed in this article.

I'm not a medical doctor and I'm not offering medical advice; I'm simply providing you with a list of tried and true supplements to help you achieve your aesthetic goal of superhero ab muscles.

Here's a caveat: The effectiveness of these supplements is increased by 100% when you use them as an ADDITION to a properly designed Eating Plan, cardiovascular and resistance training program, NOT as a replacement. Put in the work and see the results. If you're using these as a replacement, be prepared have some very expensive urine and diminished gains as a result.

In addition, many people reading this may be wondering if it's possible to get all these nutrients from food alone, and the answer is yes... IF you have the time to sit down and consume the amounts of food required to receive these nutrients. In this day and age, not many people have the time to do that. In addition, some people may have conditions that require them to receive certain nutrients through supplementation. To each his own, as they say. Moving swiftly on, shall we?

Here's another caveat: The effectiveness of these supplements is increased by 100% when you use them as an ADDITION to a properly designed cardiovascular and resistance training program, NOT as a replacement. Put in the work and see the results.

1) Branch Chain Amino Acids - Branch chain amino acids are composed of isoleucine, leucine, and valine. These are non-essential amino acids, meaning that they are not crucial to optimal functioning of your body. If however, your goal is to build lean muscle and burn fat, then they are essential.

BCAA'S are usually taken before a heavy resistance training session or a long slow duration cardio session, to help increase protein synthesis (read: muscle growth) and to decrease muscle catabolism, respectively. Preventing muscle catabolism is crucial for two reasons:

A) Abs are muscles!!

B) The less active muscle tissue you have, the higher your metabolic rate is. This means that your muscles will use more macronutrients, specifically fat, to help feed themselves.

Follow the serving size recommendation on the label when you purchase them for best results.

2) Whey Protein - Muscles are made up of ingested proteins which are broken down into amino acids, which are then synthesized into rock hard, terminator-like muscle (depending on your resistance training program). One of the cool things about whey protein is that there is very little fat or fiber, which causes your body to absorb it rather quickly once you ingest it, allowing you to take advantage of that crucial muscle rebuilding window brought on by your weight training session. To take full advantage of your whey protein supplement:

A) Make sure that you know your current body fat levels. Once you know those levels, you can determine your lean body mass and from that point; you can set a goal as to how much muscle you want to gain.

Because whey protein is absorbed so quickly, this means that it is also passed quickly through your digestive tract, meaning that you won't stay full long. Because of this property, your best bet is to use your whey protein immediately AFTER your workout. If you want to turn your whey protein into a meal, you'd have to add fats and carbohydrates to the mix.

3) Omega 3 fatty acids - These have many health benefits aside from helping your body burn fat and build more muscle easier. In addition to helping to raise your good cholesterol and reduce inflammation, Omega 3's help your body do a few amazing things, two of which are increasing insulin sensitivity and increasing your bodies' ability to uptake and absorb/utilize protein.

Increased insulin sensitivity is awesome because it means that your bodies' cells are able to uptake insulin along with glucose into your cells so that you can use them for energy like your body is supposed to. Excess insulin floating in your bloodstream can cause your body to shift into fat storing mode and can set susceptible persons up for type 2 diabetes.

Because of omega 3's ability to increase protein synthesis, this translates to less wasted protein and faster muscle gains. This supplement is a must have if you're truly serious about making lean gains fast and safely.

4) Caffeine - While I'm not a fan of so called "fat burning" supplements, I am a fan of supplements with the proper dosage of caffeine. Caffeine has been tested repeatedly and has been found to increase alertness, enhance carbohydrate utilization, and increase pain tolerance, among other benefits.

With the increase in pain tolerance, you can work harder during your training sessions and burn more calories and make more gains.

With the increased carbohydrate utilization effect, you provide another "drain" for your body to send carbohydrates down, so that your insulin levels can remain stable as you train.

With the increase in alertness caffeine provides, you minimize your chances of injuring yourself due to...well, not being alert.

If you've never used caffeine before, please check with your doctor and use LESS than the recommended serving size on your first try. If it calls for you to use 2 scoops, use 1 or even a half and increase the dosage until your determine a dosage that will let you train and not have your hearty explode in your chest.

One of the best places to get caffeine is from Green Tea. Not only does it have theanine which helps you to relax, but it has moderate levels of caffeine that are perfect for people who can't tolerate the high does usually found in coffee. It's also much gentler on your stomach.

5) L- carnitine: This amino acid is a staple of bodybuilders who want to get cut and lean fast, and now you can use it to achieve a

similar physique. L- Carnitine helps reduce your body fat levels by enhancing your cells ability to uptake long chain fatty acids and use them for energy. Long chain fatty acids are just that: really long chains of fatty acids. Fatty acid chains can be extremely hard to break down (depending on genetics, etc) in preparation to be used for energy, thus the benefits of carnitine are needed.

While you can purchase carnitine by itself, your best bet is to find a supplement that contains the Branch Chain Amino Acids in addition to carnitine. These combined amino acids will help pack a powerful fat burning punch.

6) Vitamin C- This supplement is crucial to keep in your muscle-building cabinet, however probably not for the reasons you may be thinking. Vitamin c helps our bodies deal with stress more effectively. When we get stressed out, our bodies' release varying levels of cortisol. Cortisol in healthy amounts helps us deal with stress, but when the cortisol levels in your body are high, some very awful things start to take place:

A) Your body starts to break down that sweet, sweet muscle tissue to be used for energy.

B) Your body starts to store fat.

That's a depressing double whammy to your gains, isn't it?

Keeping your vitamin c levels at a good place in your body will help you deal with the stress in your daily life better and the stress of working out.

7) Beta Alanine- This is a awesome supplement if your training program is composed of lots of resistance training. Beta Alanine helps your body to perform more reps before you get to fatigue. With the right training program, you can see huge gains in lean muscle tissue and strength output.

There are two things that most people don't like about the supplement:

A) The annoying itchy feeling that can accompany its use.

B) The fact that you have to take it daily to see results.

If you can get past these two factors, you'll be one step closer to gigantic, robotic ab muscles.

8) Creatine - Tried and tested for decades now, creatine is another supplement you must have to achieve your full muscular and athletic potential. Creatine works by causing you muscles to hold more water. Since water carries nutrients to your cells, higher water storage means that you can get more nutrients to the muscles, and thus squeeze out more reps before fatigue.

Use the recommended serving size to avoid excess water storage.

9) Multivitamin - A good multivitamin will provide your with all the vitamins and minerals you need to make sure that your muscles grow as planned. Some of the key muscle building ingredients in a multivitamin are Zinc and Vitamin D (which is actually a hormone), both of which help to increase your testosterone levels, which in

turn helps increase lean muscle mass. Your best bet is to get a "2 a day" multivitamin, taking one pill/dose in the morning and one in the evening, depending on how long your days are and how active you are.

10) Milk Thistle: Now, this supplement can be considered optional. However, if you can afford it, add it to your muscle building supplement stack. Milk thistle helps your liver to burn fat better; it also helps your liver to process estrogen better. This is crucial if you're a man wanting to build and maintain lean muscle mass. Excess estrogen in your blood stream can contribute to decreased free testosterone and gynecomastia, which is enlargement of male breast tissue.

Keep in mind that these supplements are to be used IN CONJUNCTION a balanced diet of lean proteins/ vegetable proteins, complex carbohydrates, and healthy fats like avocados and nuts.

Appendix 3

Seasonal supplements for Stress Support and immune health

Even if you don't live in a climate that gets nice and dreary for 5 months out of the year, you still need support for your immune system. You need this support even more if you work with lots of people and in closed spaces.

Here are several powerful supplements to help you boost your immune system and increase your energy levels naturally:

1) <u>Probiotics</u> – This may come as a shock to a lot of you reading this now, but a major portion of your immune system lies in your gut. About 75% to be exact. Having a good balance of good bacteria and bad bacteria is crucial to maintaining not only proper digestive health, but optimal immune system health and high energy levels.

2) <u>Ginseng</u> – this is one herb most of you may have heard of, possibly spoken of only in whispers and hushes. Ginseng herb falls in the category of Adaptogens, meaning that they have compounds that help your body to adapt to stressful situations easier. Less stress means less cortisol production, which means more energy and vitality!

3) <u>Reishi mushroom</u> – This mushroom has compounds that strengthen your immune system to keep it humming strong and powerful.

4) <u>Goldenseal</u> – this herb is a powerful antibiotic.

5) <u>Rhodiola</u> Extract – this herbs boosts your immune system, helps increases your energy levels, and makes sex more enjoyable.

Appendix 4

Additional resources for Success!

Check out my Youtube Channel for additional FREE resources on health, fitness, and peak performance:

https://www.youtube.com/channel/UCVJbxyOzfSMQY9JWUYGQ82A

In addition, I am available for speaking engagements and group peak performance trainings. Please contact me at masterkeyshealth@gmail.com for more details.

For updates and free peak performance info, subscribe to my blog now and get in on the action:

https://seathebiggerpicture.wordpress.com/

Stay in the loop, and stay Growing Better!!

www.ingramcontent.com/pod-product-compliance
Lightning Source LLC
Chambersburg PA
CBHW081344280526
45788CB00009B/2771